SUZANNE BYRD

# Borderline & Beyond

*A Guide for Women with BPD*

# Contents

1   Introduction – A Journey of Understanding      1

2   The Landscape of Borderline Personality Disorder
in Women      8

3   Unraveling the Roots – Early Experiences and Identity...      16

4   Stigma, Misunderstanding, and the Fight for Self-Acceptance      24

5   Introduction to DBT and Other Coping Tools      33

6   Deep Dive into Mindfulness and Emotional Regulation      43

7   Building and Maintaining Healthy Relationships      52

8   Rediscovering and Embracing Your Identity      62

9   Healing Through Narrative – The Power of Personal Stories      72

10   Building a Support Network – Finding Allies and Mentors      82

11   Tools for Transformation – Empowerment Strategies and...      90

12   Beyond the Diagnosis – Embracing a Life of Authenticity and...      98

# 1

# Introduction – A Journey of Understanding

Borderline Personality Disorder (BPD) is a complex, often misunder-stood condition that affects many women. In this opening chapter, we embark on a journey of understanding—a journey that is as much about personal discovery as it is about unpacking clinical insights and societal narratives. This book, Borderline & Beyond: A Guide for Women with BPD, is both a memoir and a self-help guide. It draws on lived experience, clinical tools, and the wisdom found in other influential works such as Girl, Interrupted by Susanna Kaysen, I Hate You, Don't Leave Me by Jerold J. Kreisman and Hal Straus, and The Dialectical Behavior Therapy Skills Workbook by McKay, Wood, and Brantley. These texts have paved the way for understanding mental health struggles, and their perspectives offer valuable context for the discussions that follow.

## Embracing the Complexity of BPD

When I first encountered the diagnosis of BPD, it felt as though I had been handed a label that was both confusing and stigmatizing. Society often paints BPD with broad, negative strokes—a condition marked solely by chaos, instability, and emotional extremes. However, as I grew to understand my own experiences and listened to the stories of other women living with BPD, I discovered that beneath the surface of intense emotions lay a vibrant complexity, a tapestry of resilience, creativity, and depth. This realization is at the heart of this book.

Understanding BPD begins with acknowledging its dual nature. It is a disorder that brings great challenges—fear of abandonment, impulsivity, and overwhelming emotional turmoil—yet it also endows those who live with it with heightened sensitivity and empathy. This paradox is something many authors have explored over the years. In *Girl, Interrupted*, Susanna Kaysen provides a candid and deeply personal account of life within the confines of mental health institutions, revealing the hidden layers of humanity that can reside even in those deemed "unwell." Similarly, *I Hate You, Don't Leave Me* delves into the tumultuous relationships and internal battles characteristic of BPD, offering readers both a clinical perspective and a compassionate understanding of the disorder.

## A Hybrid Approach: Memoir Meets Self-Help

This book is designed to be a companion for every woman who has ever felt isolated by her diagnosis. It is structured as a hybrid—merging memoir with practical self-help strategies. I share my own story: the struggles, the setbacks, and the small victories. Alongside personal narratives, you will find guidance on Dialectical Behavior Therapy (DBT) skills, mindfulness practices, and other coping tools that have helped me navigate the stormy waters of BPD. The goal is not only to provide validation for your feelings but also to offer concrete strategies that can help you take control of your emotional life.

The journey outlined in this chapter is the first step towards reclaiming your narrative. Like many women before us, I once felt trapped in a cycle of self-doubt and misunderstanding—a cycle perpetuated by both internal fears and external judgments. Over time, however, I learned that while BPD is a significant part of my identity, it does not define the totality of who I am. This realization is echoed in many self-help guides that encourage a redefinition of self beyond labels. Books like *The Dialectical Behavior Therapy Skills Workbook* provide structured exercises that not only help manage symptoms but also encourage an exploration of self-identity outside the confines of a diagnosis.

## The Stigma and the Silence

One of the most painful aspects of living with BPD is the stigma that surrounds it. Society often reduces complex emotional experiences to simple stereotypes, labeling women with BPD as "difficult" or "manipulative." This stigma is further compounded by a lack of understanding from both the public and, at times, even mental health professionals. For many years, the conversation about BPD was shrouded in silence, with those affected feeling isolated and ashamed. Breaking this silence is crucial.

In sharing my own story, I hope to foster a sense of community and understanding. I want to show that there is power in vulnerability and that by opening up about our experiences, we can begin to dismantle the misconceptions that surround BPD. In doing so, we pave the way for a more nuanced conversation about mental health—one that recognizes the individuality of each experience rather than reducing it to a set of symptoms. This approach is reminiscent of the transformative narratives found in books like *Girl, Interrupted*, where personal reflection and storytelling become instruments for both healing and empowerment.

## The Role of Research and Personal Experience

Scientific research has long identified that a significant majority of those diagnosed with BPD are women. This statistic is not merely a number—it represents real lives, each with its own story of struggle and triumph. The clinical literature provides us with frameworks to understand the symptoms and challenges associated with BPD, yet it is the personal stories behind these frameworks that add depth and humanity to the conversation. I draw upon both scientific research and my own experiences, blending them to create a resource that is at once informative and deeply personal.

For instance, the integration of DBT skills into daily life has been a game changer for me. DBT, with its focus on mindfulness, emotional regulation, and interpersonal effectiveness, offers practical tools to manage the chaos that often accompanies BPD. As you explore the chapters ahead, you will encounter detailed explanations and exercises inspired by works such as *The Dialectical Behavior Therapy Skills Workbook*. This practical approach not only demystifies the therapeutic process but also empowers you to take an active role in your own healing journey.

## Laying the Groundwork for a New Narrative

The purpose of this book is not to provide a one-size-fits-all solution but rather to offer a roadmap for crafting your own narrative—a narrative where BPD is acknowledged, understood, and ultimately integrated into a broader story of growth and resilience. In these pages, you will find both scientific explanations and personal reflections. This dual approach is designed to help you see that while BPD is a challenge, it is also a source of strength.

The idea of embracing a "new narrative" is inspired by other transformative works. For example, *I Hate You, Don't Leave Me* not only explains the clinical aspects of BPD but also invites readers to reflect on how societal expectations shape our understanding of mental illness. By integrating these perspectives, you are encouraged to question the status quo and to redefine what it means to live with BPD. It's about recognizing that the same sensitivity which can lead to emotional overwhelm is also the wellspring of creativity, empathy, and deep personal insight.

## A Personal Invitation

I invite you to join me on this journey—a journey that will explore the intricacies of BPD and celebrate the resilience that lies within each of us. Whether you are someone living with BPD or a loved one seeking to understand, this book is written with you in mind. It is a testament to the power of sharing our stories and the importance of building communities where we support one another in our struggles and triumphs.

Throughout my own journey, I encountered numerous setbacks. There were moments when I felt utterly alone, burdened by the weight of societal judgment and internal self-criticism. Yet, it was in these moments of darkness that I discovered the seeds of transformation. By learning to apply DBT skills and embracing the power of mindfulness, I began to see my experiences in a new light—not as a life sentence defined by disorder, but as a chapter in a much larger story of growth and self-discovery.

## Connecting with Other Voices

In many ways, this book is also a conversation—a dialogue between the experiences of countless women who have walked similar paths. The stories and insights of others, as shared in books like *Girl, Interrupted* and *I Hate You, Don't Leave Me*, have been invaluable in shaping my understanding of BPD. These works have shown that even when the world seems to be stacked against you, there is a way forward—a way to transform pain into power and struggle into strength.

As you progress through the chapters, you will find that this book is not just about managing a disorder but about reclaiming your voice and redefining your identity. It is an invitation to explore the layers of your personality and to recognize that your emotional depth is not a flaw to be hidden, but a gift to be understood and nurtured.

## Setting the Stage for Healing

Healing from BPD is not a linear process—it is a journey filled with peaks and valleys, triumphs and setbacks. There will be times when the skills you learn seem to fall short, and moments when old habits resurface. Yet, each step you take is a testament to your resilience and determination. This book is structured to support you through those ups and downs, offering practical tools and reflective narratives that you can return to time and again.

As we move forward, I encourage you to approach this journey with an open heart and a willingness to experiment with new ways of thinking and being. Embrace the tools offered here not as rigid prescriptions but as flexible guidelines that you can adapt to your own needs. Remember, the path to healing is uniquely personal, and every small victory is a milestone worth celebrating.

## A Glimpse of What Lies Ahead

In the chapters that follow, we will delve deeper into topics such as the origins of BPD, the role of early experiences in shaping identity, and the transformative power of mindfulness and DBT skills. We will explore how to build healthier relationships, develop a supportive network, and ultimately redefine what it means to live beyond the diagnosis. Each chapter builds on the last, creating a comprehensive guide that is as empathetic as it is practical.

This introduction is merely the beginning—a call to start looking at BPD not as an endless battle, but as a part of your multifaceted identity. It is an invitation to question the conventional wisdom surrounding mental health and to discover the inner strength that has always been there, waiting to be acknowledged.

As you turn the page and embark on this journey with me, remember that you are not alone. The experiences shared in this book are drawn from my own life and the lives of countless other women who have learned to navigate the complexities of BPD. Together, we will challenge stigma, celebrate our strengths, and forge a path toward a more compassionate, empowered future.

Let this book be a trusted companion on your journey—a guide that provides not only practical tools but also the comfort of knowing that your struggles are seen, understood, and valued. Welcome to a journey of understanding, healing, and ultimately, transformation.

In the coming chapters, we will explore the intricacies of Borderline Personality Disorder with the same honesty and compassion that characterize this introduction. With references to influential works and practical self-help strategies, we are setting the stage for a new narrative—one that honors your unique experience and celebrates your potential for growth.

# 2

# The Landscape of Borderline Personality Disorder in Women

Borderline Personality Disorder (BPD) is a multifaceted and often misunderstood condition, and its prevalence among women adds a layer of complexity to its narrative. In this chapter, we explore the social, historical, and clinical landscape of BPD, with a particular focus on how the disorder affects women. By examining research, societal perceptions, and personal accounts, we aim to create a richer understanding of the dynamics at play. Throughout this discussion, I will reference influential works that have shaped our understanding of BPD, such as Girl, Interrupted by Susanna Kaysen, I Hate You, Don't Leave Me by Jerold J. Kreisman and Hal Straus, and The Dialectical Behavior Therapy Skills Workbook by McKay, Wood, and Brantley.

## The Gendered Diagnosis: Why Women?

A striking aspect of BPD is that approximately 75% of those diagnosed are women. This statistic raises an important question: why are women more likely to receive this diagnosis? Several factors come into play, ranging from biological and psychological differences to cultural expectations and gender biases in mental health care. Critics argue that diagnostic criteria have historically been influenced by gendered stereotypes, often labeling behaviors in women as pathological when they might be understood differently in men.

In *Girl, Interrupted*, Susanna Kaysen presents a narrative that delves into the gendered nuances of mental illness. Her memoir illustrates how societal expectations and the clinical environment can conspire to produce a diagnosis that carries both a clinical label and a social stigma. The tendency to pathologize emotional expressiveness and relational dependency in women contributes significantly to the high prevalence of BPD diagnoses among them.

Furthermore, *I Hate You, Don't Leave Me* offers an in-depth look at the emotional turbulence and interpersonal challenges that often accompany BPD. The book underscores how the behaviors associated with the disorder are frequently interpreted through a gendered lens. For example, what might be seen as assertiveness or independence in one context may be misinterpreted as instability or manipulation when exhibited by a woman. This misinterpretation further complicates the way women experience and are treated for BPD.

## Societal Narratives and Cultural Expectations

Women have long been subject to societal expectations that demand emotional labor, selflessness, and stability—qualities that are often at odds with the experiences of those living with BPD. Cultural narratives can paint women as inherently nurturing and emotionally resilient, making it all the more challenging for those with BPD to be understood and accepted. When women deviate from these idealized roles, their behavior may be met with harsh judgment rather than empathy.

This disconnect between societal expectations and the reality of living with BPD contributes to the stigma surrounding the disorder. Books like *Girl, Interrupted* and *I Hate You, Don't Leave Me* have played pivotal roles in shedding light on these cultural tensions. They reveal how the struggle for self-identity, autonomy, and emotional validation is often exacerbated by societal pressures. In this light, BPD is not simply a medical diagnosis but a reflection of deeper cultural conflicts about gender, power, and identity.

The cultural narrative often isolates women who do not conform to traditional roles. This isolation can result in a profound sense of shame and self-blame, making it even more difficult for individuals to seek help. As we explore this landscape, it becomes clear that understanding BPD in women requires us to challenge and reframe these entrenched societal narratives.

## The Historical Evolution of BPD

Historically, the conceptualization of BPD has evolved significantly. Early descriptions of the disorder were often entangled with psychoanalytic theories that placed undue emphasis on early childhood experiences and dysfunctional family dynamics. Over time, the diagnostic criteria have been refined to focus more on the observable symptoms and behaviors associated with emotional dysregulation and unstable interpersonal relationships.

The evolution of BPD as a diagnostic category has not been without controversy. Many critics argue that the criteria have been overly influenced by gendered biases, which has led to an overdiagnosis in women. This critique is explored in depth in *I Hate You, Don't Leave Me*, where the authors examine how early mental health paradigms often misinterpreted the emotional lives of women. The book discusses how behaviors such as intense emotional expression and dependency were once dismissed as mere hysteria or neurosis, only to be reinterpreted later as symptoms of a more specific disorder.

While modern diagnostic tools have improved our ability to understand BPD, remnants of these historical biases continue to influence clinical practice. Awareness of this history is crucial for both clinicians and those living with BPD, as it informs a more compassionate and accurate understanding of the disorder. This chapter, therefore, not only examines current perspectives but also acknowledges the historical context that has shaped the modern landscape of BPD diagnosis and treatment.

## The Clinical Picture: Symptoms and Challenges

From a clinical standpoint, BPD is characterized by a pervasive pattern of instability in interpersonal relationships, self-image, and affect, as well as marked impulsivity. These symptoms can manifest in a variety of ways, such as rapid mood swings, fear of abandonment, self-destructive behaviors, and difficulties in maintaining stable relationships. The complexity of these symptoms often leads to misdiagnosis and misunderstanding.

In *The Dialectical Behavior Therapy Skills Workbook*, McKay, Wood, and Brantley offer practical insights into the coping mechanisms that can be applied to manage these symptoms. DBT is particularly effective in helping individuals develop mindfulness, emotional regulation, distress tolerance, and interpersonal effectiveness—skills that are essential for navigating the challenges of BPD. The workbook provides not only exercises and strategies but also a framework for understanding how these skills can transform day-to-day experiences.

Clinically, the challenges of BPD are compounded by the fact that the symptoms can be both self-perpetuating and externally influenced. For example, the intense fear of abandonment may lead to behaviors that inadvertently push loved ones away, thus reinforcing the individual's worst fears. Similarly, the impulsivity that characterizes BPD can result in actions that have long-term negative consequences, further entrenching the cycle of emotional instability.

This cyclical nature of symptoms is a core aspect of the disorder. Recognizing these patterns is the first step toward developing effective coping strategies. In the pages that follow, we will explore how practical tools, such as those offered in DBT, can help break these cycles and foster a more stable, empowered way of living.

## The Intersection of Biology and Environment

Understanding the landscape of BPD requires an examination of the interplay between biological predispositions and environmental influences. Research suggests that genetic factors may contribute to a susceptibility to emotional dysregulation, but environmental factors—such as early childhood experiences, trauma, and family dynamics—play a significant role in triggering and shaping the disorder.

The dual influence of nature and nurture is a recurring theme in discussions of BPD. The sensitivity that often characterizes individuals with BPD may be rooted in their biological makeup, but it is the environment in which that sensitivity is nurtured—or neglected—that determines how it manifests. Books like *Girl, Interrupted* provide poignant insights into how external circumstances, including the treatment received from family and society, can exacerbate the vulnerabilities inherent in the disorder.

Moreover, environmental stressors such as societal expectations, relationship conflicts, and economic hardships can compound the difficulties experienced by women with BPD. These external pressures often intensify the internal struggle, creating a feedback loop that can be hard to break. The challenge, then, is not only to address the symptoms of BPD but also to navigate the broader context in which these symptoms occur.

## A Call for Compassionate Understanding

As we traverse the landscape of BPD, it is essential to emphasize the need for a compassionate, nuanced approach to both diagnosis and treatment. Too often, the emotional experiences of women with BPD are dismissed or oversimplified. In reality, these experiences are multifaceted, influenced by a range of biological, psychological, and cultural factors.

The works referenced in this chapter—*Girl, Interrupted, I Hate You, Don't Leave Me*, and *The Dialectical Behavior Therapy Skills Workbook*—all advocate for a deeper, more empathetic understanding of BPD. They challenge the reductionist view that sees BPD merely as a collection of symptoms and instead present it as a complex interplay of factors that deserve careful consideration. By integrating these perspectives, we can begin to dismantle the stigma that surrounds the disorder and foster an environment in which women feel seen, heard, and supported.

A compassionate approach means acknowledging the full humanity of those with BPD. It means validating their experiences, recognizing their struggles, and celebrating their resilience. It is about understanding that the emotional intensity associated with BPD, while challenging, is also a source of creativity, empathy, and profound personal insight. This reframing of the narrative is crucial for transforming how society views and treats BPD.

## Moving Forward: Integrating Knowledge and Empathy

In this chapter, we have navigated the broad landscape of Borderline Personality Disorder in women by exploring the gendered aspects of diagnosis, the impact of cultural expectations, the historical evolution of clinical perspectives, and the intricate interplay of biological and environmental factors. Each of these elements contributes to the complex picture of BPD, highlighting both the challenges and the potential for growth.

As we move forward in this book, we will delve deeper into the personal and practical aspects of living with BPD. Future chapters will offer insights into coping strategies, such as mindfulness and DBT, as well as tools for building healthier relationships and reclaiming personal identity. The knowledge shared in this chapter lays the groundwork for understanding the roots of BPD and the multifaceted influences that shape its manifestation in women.

Ultimately, this exploration is a call to action: a call for both individuals and society to recognize the need for compassionate, informed approaches to mental health. The stories and research shared here are not just academic—they are lived experiences that offer a roadmap for understanding and healing. By embracing this comprehensive perspective, we can work together to create a future where women with BPD are not defined by their diagnosis but empowered by the strength, insight, and resilience that lie within them.

In drawing on the narratives and insights of influential works such as *Girl, Interrupted*, *I Hate You, Don't Leave Me*, and *The Dialectical Behavior Therapy Skills Workbook*, this chapter has aimed to illuminate the diverse factors that contribute to the experience of BPD in women. These references remind us that while the clinical aspects of BPD are important, so too are the personal stories and cultural contexts that shape how the disorder is experienced and understood.

As you reflect on the material presented in this chapter, I invite you to consider the broader implications of these insights—not only for those living with BPD but for all of us who seek to understand the complexities of human emotion and behavior. The journey toward compassionate understanding begins with acknowledging the rich tapestry of experiences that define what it means to live with BPD, and it is my hope that this chapter serves as both an educational resource and a source of empowerment for every reader.

Let us now continue this journey together, armed with knowledge, empathy, and the belief that understanding the landscape of BPD is the first step toward creating a more inclusive and supportive world for women everywhere.

# 3

# Unraveling the Roots – Early Experiences and Identity Formation

The journey of understanding oneself often begins long before we can consciously articulate our struggles. For many women with Borderline Personality Disorder (BPD), the roots of the condition are deeply intertwined with early experiences, family dynamics, and cultural influences. In this chapter, we will explore how early life events shape identity formation, impact emotional regulation, and set the stage for the challenges—and strengths—that later emerge. Through personal narrative, clinical insights, and reflective exercises, this chapter aims to help you unravel the threads of your past to better understand who you are today.

## The Imprint of Early Experiences

Our earliest experiences leave indelible marks on our emotional and psychological development. In childhood, we learn how to navigate the world through the lens of our relationships, primarily with our caregivers. These formative interactions set patterns for how we view ourselves and others, influencing our sense of safety, trust, and self-worth.

For many women with BPD, early life experiences may have included inconsistent caregiving, experiences of abandonment, or environments where emotions were either neglected or overly dramatized. When a child does not receive a stable, secure foundation, the brain's natural development of emotional regulation and self-identity can be disrupted. The result may be a heightened sensitivity to perceived rejection and a tendency toward intense emotional responses.

Reflecting on my own childhood, I recall moments when the line between love and fear was blurred. There were instances of unpredictability—times when a loving embrace could quickly turn into silence or anger. Over time, these experiences taught me to hyper-attune to the emotional cues around me, a survival mechanism that later manifested as the intense relational dynamics characteristic of BPD.

## Family Dynamics and the Formation of Self

Family is often our first social network, and the dynamics within our family can shape our identity in powerful ways. In families where emotional expression was met with criticism, dismissal, or even punishment, a child might learn to suppress their feelings or, conversely, express them in extreme ways in order to be heard. This dichotomy can create a confusing internal landscape where the child is unsure which part of their emotional self is "acceptable."

Consider the way that family roles are assigned, sometimes unconsciously. One child might be cast as the "responsible one" while another might be labeled as the "sensitive" or "troubled" child. In many cases, women with BPD have internalized the role of the "emotional caretaker" or have been unfairly burdened with expectations that they must manage not only their own feelings but also the emotions of those around them. These roles, often rigidly defined in the family structure, can restrict personal growth and lead to an identity that is overly entwined with the needs and moods of others.

It is important to recognize that these early patterns are not a personal failing. They are adaptations to an environment that may have been lacking in consistency or emotional safety. Understanding this context allows for a compassionate view of oneself, paving the way for healing and growth.

## Cultural Influences and the Narrative of Self

Beyond the family unit, cultural influences also play a crucial role in shaping our identity. Society often prescribes rigid gender roles that can affect how women experience and express their emotions. In many cultures, women are expected to be the nurturers, the empathizers, and the keepers of social harmony. When a woman's emotional experiences deviate from these expectations—whether through intensity or unpredictability—it can lead to feelings of inadequacy or guilt.

From a young age, many women are taught that vulnerability is a weakness rather than a strength. This societal pressure to conform to an idealized image of emotional restraint can be particularly damaging for those who naturally experience emotions in a more expansive, intense manner. When cultural expectations clash with personal experiences, the result can be an internal conflict that challenges the very core of one's identity.

I have often found myself questioning the origin of these cultural expectations. Were the intense emotions I experienced a personal flaw, or were they a natural response to a world that demanded restraint? Over time, I have come to see that the emotional intensity associated with BPD is not a weakness, but a form of sensitivity that has its own unique strengths—such as empathy, creativity, and resilience. This realization has been liberating, allowing me to redefine my identity beyond the limitations imposed by external expectations.

## The Journey Toward Understanding: Personal Reflections

In my own journey, coming to terms with early experiences was both painful and transformative. I began to see that many of the patterns that once felt like traps were, in fact, survival strategies honed in response to an unpredictable world. For example, I learned that my hypervigilance in relationships was not a defect but a learned behavior designed to anticipate and mitigate the pain of abandonment.

Journaling became a critical tool for me—a way to trace the origins of my emotional responses back to specific memories and relationships. By writing about my childhood experiences, I gradually uncovered recurring themes: the longing for stability, the need for validation, and the struggle to separate my identity from the emotions of those around me. This process was not always easy, as it forced me to confront painful truths about my past. However, it was also profoundly liberating. I began to see that my experiences, while difficult, had also endowed me with a depth of understanding and a capacity for compassion that I might not have otherwise developed.

Through these reflections, I started to appreciate that every experience, every relationship, had contributed to the person I am today. The process of understanding my early experiences was akin to piecing together a mosaic—each shard, no matter how jagged, played a role in creating a larger, more intricate picture of my identity.

## The Role of Therapy in Unraveling the Past

While personal reflection is invaluable, professional guidance can also be instrumental in untangling the complex web of early experiences and identity formation. Therapy, particularly approaches such as

Dialectical Behavior Therapy (DBT) and psychodynamic therapy, offers structured ways to explore these formative years. DBT, for instance, helps individuals develop mindfulness and emotional regulation skills that are essential for navigating the turbulent waters of early emotional trauma.

In my sessions with a compassionate therapist, I learned how to identify triggers that were directly linked to past experiences. Together, we worked on strategies to ground myself in the present while gently unpacking the past. These therapeutic techniques were crucial in helping me separate the person I was becoming from the pain of what I had experienced. Therapy provided a safe space to confront the parts of myself that had been shaped by early instability, allowing me to reclaim those parts and integrate them into a coherent, empowered self-identity.

## Rediscovering Identity Beyond the Diagnosis

One of the most empowering aspects of this journey is the realization that while early experiences shape us, they do not have to define us. Understanding the roots of our emotional patterns can lead to a profound transformation in how we view ourselves. This process is not about erasing the past but about integrating it into a broader narrative of growth and resilience.

I have learned that identity is not static. It is fluid, continuously evolving as we accumulate new experiences and insights. The challenge—and the beauty—of life is that we have the power to rewrite our own stories. In embracing this fluidity, I have begun to see my sensitivity not as a defect, but as a vital part of who I am—a gift that enables me to connect deeply with others and appreciate the nuances of life.

This shift in perspective is echoed in many therapeutic and self-help frameworks. For instance, the exercises found in DBT encourage individuals to observe their thoughts and emotions without judgment, allowing for a clearer understanding of how past experiences influence present behavior. Through mindfulness and reflective practice, it becomes possible to develop a more nuanced view of one's identity—one that honors the past while making space for future growth.

## The Interplay of Nature and Nurture

In exploring early experiences, it is important to acknowledge the interplay between nature and nurture. While our environment and relationships play a significant role in shaping us, there is also a biological component to how we process emotions. Research has shown that genetic predispositions can influence emotional sensitivity and reactivity. For women with BPD, this heightened sensitivity might be both a blessing and a challenge.

Understanding that there is a biological basis for some of our experiences can be incredibly validating. It shifts the narrative away from one of personal blame and toward a more compassionate understanding of our inherent predispositions. Recognizing the dual influence of genetics and environment allows us to see that our struggles are not solely the result of a flawed upbringing, but are also part of a complex interplay of factors that contribute to our unique identity.

## Embracing the Complexity of Identity Formation

The journey of identity formation is rarely straightforward. It is a dynamic, often messy process that involves reconciling conflicting parts of ourselves. For many women with BPD, there is an ongoing tension between the desire to belong and the fear of being overwhelmed by others' expectations. This tension can manifest as a constant push and pull between dependency and autonomy, a struggle to balance intimacy with independence.

Over time, I have come to embrace this complexity as an integral part of my identity. The process of unraveling the roots of my early experiences has taught me that there is beauty in the struggle. Every moment of pain, every flash of anger, and every tear shed in isolation has contributed to the rich tapestry of who I am. This understanding has been a cornerstone of my healing process, allowing me to move forward with a sense of wholeness rather than fragmentation.

## Moving Toward Integration and Healing

As we near the end of this chapter, it is important to emphasize that unraveling the roots of our past is not about dwelling in pain—it is about using that understanding as a foundation for healing. The insights gained from examining early experiences can inform new, healthier patterns of thought and behavior. By acknowledging the influence of our past, we can begin to integrate those experiences into a coherent narrative that supports personal growth.

Practical exercises, such as guided journaling and mindfulness meditation, can be invaluable tools in this process. I encourage you to set aside time each day to reflect on your early memories—both the painful and the joyful. As you write, try to observe your emotions without judgment. Notice any recurring themes or patterns. This practice can help you develop a compassionate perspective on your past and foster a sense of empowerment over your present and future.

## The Path to a Coherent Self

Unraveling the roots of early experiences is a profound and sometimes challenging journey. It requires courage to face the parts of ourselves that have been shaped by adversity. Yet, in this process lies the potential for profound healing and transformation. As you continue to explore your own story, remember that every experience—no matter how painful—has contributed to the unique, multifaceted person you are today.

This chapter has explored the impact of early experiences, family dynamics, and cultural influences on identity formation. It has also highlighted the importance of therapy, mindfulness, and self-reflection in understanding and integrating these early influences. By acknowledging both the hardships and the strengths that have emerged from your past, you can begin to craft a narrative of self that is resilient, compassionate, and empowered.

As you move forward in this book, carry with you the understanding that your past is not a chain that binds you, but a foundation upon which you can build a future filled with possibility and growth. Embrace the complexity of your identity, and allow your early experiences to inform— but not define—the powerful, authentic person you are becoming.

In the next chapter, we will delve further into the pervasive stigma and misunderstanding surrounding BPD, exploring how societal narratives have shaped our internal worlds. By continuing this journey of self-discovery and understanding, you will be better equipped to challenge those narratives and build a life that honors the entirety of your experience.

Remember, the process of unearthing and understanding your early experiences is not linear—it is a winding path filled with both setbacks and breakthroughs. Each step you take is a testament to your resilience and a stride toward a more coherent, integrated sense of self. Embrace this journey with compassion, and know that each moment of reflection brings you closer to the empowered identity you deserve to claim.

# 4

# Stigma, Misunderstanding, and the Fight for Self-Acceptance

Living with Borderline Personality Disorder (BPD) often means carrying not only the weight of internal struggles but also the burden of external judgment. Stigma—the negative stereotypes and prejudices associated with mental illness—can deeply impact self-esteem and the willingness to seek help. In this chapter, we delve into how stigma and misunderstanding shape the lives of women with BPD, explore the roots of these societal attitudes, and provide strategies for fighting back through self-acceptance and empowerment.

## The Heavy Burden of Stigma

For many, the diagnosis of BPD comes as a shock, compounded by the harsh labels that society has long attached to the condition. Women with BPD are frequently painted as "manipulative," "unstable," or "overly emotional," labels that not only misrepresent the true nature of the disorder but also contribute to self-doubt and isolation. These stereotypes can be pervasive in everyday interactions—whether in casual conversations, workplace dynamics, or even within the healthcare system itself.

I recall moments when a diagnosis, intended as a pathway to healing, instead felt like a scarlet letter. The weight of judgment made me question my worth and my identity. The cultural narrative often suggests that emotional sensitivity is a flaw, rather than the rich, nuanced trait it can be. Works like *Girl, Interrupted* by Susanna Kaysen have shown how easily society can misinterpret the emotional intensity of those with BPD, reinforcing negative self-images. Such portrayals contribute to an environment where vulnerability is met with disdain, and the struggle for self-acceptance becomes even more daunting.

## Internalizing Misunderstanding

When society repeatedly bombards us with negative stereotypes, it is easy to internalize these messages. Internalized stigma can lead to feelings of shame, self-blame, and the belief that one's emotional pain is a personal failing. This internal conflict creates a vicious cycle: the more one believes the harmful messages, the more isolated and unworthy one feels, making it even harder to reach out for support or to embrace a more compassionate view of oneself.

In my own experience, I often felt trapped between two opposing forces: the urge to hide my true self to avoid criticism, and the longing to be authentic. The fear of rejection—stemming from both past experiences and cultural narratives—forced me into a pattern of self-silencing. I learned to mask my true emotions, afraid that any display of intensity would be met with misunderstanding or outright hostility.

This internal struggle is not unique. *I Hate You, Don't Leave Me* by Jerold J. Kreisman and Hal Straus poignantly captures how individuals with BPD can become ensnared in a cycle of self-doubt, where every emotional outburst is seen as evidence of personal inadequacy rather than a natural expression of a deeply sensitive inner world. The constant battle to reconcile one's internal reality with external expectations can lead to profound feelings of isolation and despair.

## Challenging Cultural Narratives

The negative stereotypes associated with BPD are not formed in a vacuum. They are the product of long-standing cultural narratives that equate emotional volatility with moral or personal failure. Women, in particular, are expected to embody grace, stability, and emotional balance. When these expectations are not met, the result is often harsh criticism and marginalization.

The media and popular culture have played significant roles in reinforcing these harmful narratives. Television shows, movies, and even news stories frequently portray individuals with BPD in a negative light, focusing on dramatic behaviors rather than the complex human experiences underlying them. This portrayal not only misrepresents the disorder but also perpetuates a cycle of misunderstanding that makes it difficult for those affected to advocate for themselves.

However, there is a growing movement to challenge these narratives. Mental health advocates and authors are increasingly using their platforms to shed light on the true nature of BPD—emphasizing its complexity, the resilience it can foster, and the unique strengths it may bring. Books like *The Dialectical Behavior Therapy Skills Workbook* by McKay, Wood, and Brantley have empowered countless individuals by offering concrete strategies to manage symptoms, all while validating the emotional depth and lived experiences of those with the disorder.

## The Fight for Self-Acceptance

Despite the external pressures and internalized negativity, the fight for self-acceptance is possible. Self-acceptance does not mean resigning oneself to the label of BPD; rather, it is about acknowledging every part of oneself—the strengths, the struggles, and the inherent worth that exists independent of any diagnosis.

One of the most transformative aspects of my own journey has been learning to reframe my experiences. Rather than viewing my emotional intensity as a liability, I gradually began to see it as a source of insight, creativity, and deep empathy. This reframing process was neither immediate nor easy; it required a deliberate and sustained effort to counteract the negative messages ingrained over years of misunderstanding.

In practical terms, self-acceptance involves both internal work and external action. On a personal level, mindfulness practices and journaling can help individuals develop a kinder, more compassionate inner dialogue. By paying attention to negative self-talk and challenging it with evidence of personal strength and resilience, it is possible to begin dismantling the harmful internalized narratives that have long defined one's self-image.

Engaging in therapy can also be transformative. Dialectical Behavior Therapy (DBT), for example, offers tools specifically designed to help individuals regulate their emotions and develop a more balanced self-perception. The structured exercises in DBT not only teach practical skills for managing distress but also promote a deeper understanding of one's emotional patterns, paving the way for genuine self-acceptance.

## Building a Supportive Community

Another critical aspect of combating stigma is building and nurturing a supportive community. When surrounded by individuals who understand and validate your experiences, the weight of stigma can begin to lift. Support groups, both online and in-person, offer a space where women with BPD can share their stories without fear of judgment. In these communities, members often find that their struggles are not isolated incidents but part of a broader, shared experience.

I have personally found solace in connecting with others who understand the unique challenges of living with BPD. These relationships have been instrumental in my journey toward self-acceptance. By sharing our experiences, we create a collective narrative that emphasizes resilience over weakness and complexity over caricature. This sense of belonging can be a powerful antidote to the isolation fostered by stigma.

Books and memoirs written by women with BPD also serve as valuable resources. They offer not only practical advice but also a reminder that you are not alone in your struggles. When I read *Girl, Interrupted*, I saw my own experiences reflected in the stories of others, which helped me realize that the stereotypes I had internalized were far removed from the truth of who I am. These narratives reinforce the idea that while BPD presents real challenges, it does not diminish the beauty and depth of the human spirit.

## Strategies for Overcoming Stigma

Overcoming the stigma of BPD involves a multifaceted approach. Here are some practical strategies that have helped me and many others reclaim our identities and build a more compassionate self-view:

1. **Educate Yourself and Others:** Knowledge is a powerful tool against

ignorance. By learning more about the scientific and clinical aspects of BPD, you can challenge the stereotypes that are often perpetuated by misinformation. Sharing accurate information with friends, family, and even healthcare providers can gradually shift the narrative. Resources like *The Dialectical Behavior Therapy Skills Workbook* provide evidence-based insights that demystify the disorder.

2. **Engage in Self-Reflection:** Journaling and mindfulness practices can help you identify and challenge negative self-talk. Reflect on moments when you felt misunderstood or judged, and consider alternative, more compassionate interpretations of those experiences. Over time, this practice can rewire your internal dialogue, replacing self-criticism with self-compassion.

3. **Seek Professional Support:** Working with a therapist who understands BPD can provide a safe space to explore and reframe your experiences. Therapists trained in DBT or psychodynamic approaches can help you process past trauma and develop strategies for managing stigma in daily life.

4. **Build a Network of Support:** Whether through support groups, online communities, or trusted friends, connecting with others who share your experiences can alleviate feelings of isolation. These networks can offer practical advice, emotional support, and a sense of belonging that is crucial for healing.

5. **Advocate for Yourself:** Self-advocacy is an essential part of the fight against stigma. This might involve speaking out about your experiences, challenging misconceptions when you encounter them, or simply asserting your right to be seen as a whole person rather than a diagnosis. By advocating for yourself, you not only empower yourself but also contribute to a broader cultural shift in how BPD is understood.

## Celebrating Resilience and Strength

At its core, the fight for self-acceptance is a celebration of resilience. Every day, women with BPD navigate a complex world that often misunderstands their emotional landscape. Yet, within that complexity lies a profound strength—a capacity for empathy, creativity, and connection that is unique and deeply valuable.

In reframing my own understanding of BPD, I have come to see that the traits often labeled as "dysfunctional" can also be sources of incredible strength. The emotional intensity that once felt like a curse is now recognized as a catalyst for deep empathy and insight. The challenges of maintaining relationships have, in many ways, honed my ability to understand others on a level that few can appreciate. This shift in perspective is not about denying the difficulties of BPD; rather, it is about embracing the full spectrum of what it means to be human.

## The Journey Continues

As we progress through this book, it becomes clear that overcoming stigma is not a destination but a journey—a process that requires continual reflection, adjustment, and growth. There will be moments when old patterns of self-doubt resurface and times when the weight of societal judgment seems unbearable. In those moments, it is essential to remember that each step taken toward self-acceptance is a victory in itself.

This chapter has sought to unpack the layers of stigma and misunderstanding that have long clouded the experience of living with BPD. We have examined how societal expectations, internalized beliefs, and historical misrepresentations have all contributed to a narrative that is as damaging as it is oversimplified. Yet, within this narrative lies the possibility for transformation—a chance to rewrite our stories in ways that honor both our struggles and our strengths.

The fight for self-acceptance is, ultimately, a fight for the right to define ourselves on our own terms. It is an act of courage to reject the narrow definitions imposed by society and to embrace the full, multifaceted nature of our identities. In challenging stigma, we not only heal ourselves but also pave the way for future generations to experience a more compassionate, informed understanding of mental health.

## Looking Forward

As you continue your journey, remember that self-acceptance is an ongoing practice. It requires patience, persistence, and a willingness to confront uncomfortable truths. The tools and strategies discussed in this chapter are meant to serve as stepping stones along your path—a path that, while fraught with challenges, is also rich with opportunities for growth and renewal.

In our next chapter, we will turn our attention to the transformative power of therapy and self-help strategies. We will explore practical approaches such as Dialectical Behavior Therapy (DBT), mindfulness practices, and other coping mechanisms that empower you to manage the emotional turbulence of BPD. With each new tool you adopt, you reclaim a part of your identity that has long been overshadowed by stigma.

## Final Reflections

Stigma may cast a long shadow over the lives of those with BPD, but it does not have to define you. In embracing your true self, with all its intensity and complexity, you assert your right to be seen, heard, and valued. The journey toward self-acceptance is a brave one—one that challenges societal norms and calls for a reevaluation of what it means to live authentically.

By understanding and addressing the roots of stigma, you take a vital step toward healing. You learn to view your emotional experiences not as burdens to be hidden but as integral components of a rich, vibrant inner world. Each moment of self-compassion, every act of self-advocacy, contributes to a larger narrative of resilience—one that celebrates the full spectrum of human emotion.

May this chapter serve as both a mirror and a window—a reflection of your struggles and a glimpse into the strength that lies within you. Embrace your journey, celebrate your victories, and know that every effort to overcome stigma is a step toward a more empowered, authentic life.

In exploring the stigma and misunderstanding surrounding BPD, we have laid the groundwork for a deeper exploration of self-help strategies in the chapters to come. The insights shared here are not merely theoretical; they are born from lived experience and a relentless pursuit of self-acceptance. As you move forward, remember that every challenge you overcome is a testament to your resilience and an affirmation of your inherent worth.

Your story is powerful. It is a story of survival, of defiance against societal expectations, and of the unyielding strength found in embracing every facet of your being. Let this chapter be a reminder that, while the world may try to define you by narrow stereotypes, you have the power to rewrite your narrative—one that honors both your vulnerabilities and your extraordinary capacity for love, creativity, and transformation.

# 5

# Introduction to DBT and Other Coping Tools

When I first encountered the concepts of Dialectical Behavior Therapy (DBT) and other coping tools, I felt as though someone had finally handed me a key to unlock a door I'd long struggled to open. DBT, developed by Marsha Linehan, is a therapeutic approach specifically designed for those who experience intense emotions and challenging interpersonal dynamics. In this chapter, we'll explore the fundamental components of DBT alongside other effective strategies, providing you with a toolbox of skills to help manage the emotional turbulence of Borderline Personality Disorder (BPD).

## The Genesis of DBT: A Response to Intensity

DBT emerged in the late 1980s as a treatment tailored for individuals whose emotional experiences seemed overwhelming and who often felt trapped by their intense reactions. At its core, DBT is a blend of cognitive-behavioral techniques with mindfulness practices, reflecting an understanding that acceptance and change can coexist. It acknowledges that while the urge to change certain behaviors is strong, there is also a critical need to accept oneself in the present moment. This dual focus has resonated deeply with many women living with BPD, offering not just a method of symptom management, but a pathway toward a more balanced and compassionate relationship with oneself.

In books like *The Dialectical Behavior Therapy Skills Workbook* by McKay, Wood, and Brantley, readers are introduced to the practical exercises and strategies that form the backbone of DBT. This resource, along with others, has helped demystify the therapeutic process and has made the core principles of DBT accessible to a broader audience.

## Core Components of DBT

DBT is built around four primary skill sets that address the challenges of BPD:

### 1. Mindfulness

Mindfulness is the cornerstone of DBT. It involves cultivating an awareness of the present moment without judgment. This practice is not about suppressing or denying your emotions, but rather observing them with curiosity and acceptance. For many women with BPD, whose emotions often feel overwhelming, mindfulness offers a pause—a moment to step back from the intensity and see the situation more clearly.

Through mindfulness, you learn to recognize patterns in your thoughts and feelings, and you can begin to understand how your reactions are influenced by past experiences. For example, if you notice that feelings of abandonment trigger a disproportionate emotional response, mindfulness helps you identify this trigger and choose a more balanced reaction. Exercises such as mindful breathing, body scans, or simply taking a moment to focus on your senses can create space between an emotional surge and a reactive behavior.

## 2. Distress Tolerance

Distress tolerance skills are designed to help you endure and survive moments of crisis without resorting to behaviors that might be harmful. Life with BPD often involves navigating periods of intense emotional distress, and in those moments, the impulse to escape or numb the pain can be overwhelming. Distress tolerance teaches you to accept and ride out these moments instead of trying to fight or suppress them.

Techniques in this area include distraction strategies, self-soothing methods, and techniques like the "TIP" skills—temperature change, intense exercise, paced breathing, and paired muscle relaxation. These strategies are not meant to resolve the underlying distress but to help you manage it long enough for more sustainable, long-term solutions to take hold.

## 3. Emotion Regulation

Emotional regulation is about understanding and managing your emotions rather than being controlled by them. Many women with BPD describe their emotional lives as a rollercoaster—where highs can be euphoric and lows devastating. Emotion regulation skills focus on identifying your emotions, understanding what triggers them, and finding ways to modify the intensity or duration of these emotional experiences.

For instance, keeping an "emotion diary" can help you track your feelings and recognize patterns over time. This practice not only increases your self-awareness but also provides concrete data that can inform therapeutic strategies. By learning to name your emotions and understand their triggers, you can gradually build a sense of control over your emotional landscape.

## 4. Interpersonal Effectiveness

Interpersonal effectiveness skills help you navigate relationships with confidence and clarity. For many women with BPD, relationships can be a source of both deep fulfillment and significant distress. Learning to communicate needs, set boundaries, and resolve conflicts without escalating emotions is essential.

These skills involve learning how to ask for what you need, say no when necessary, and manage conflicts in a healthy way. They also emphasize maintaining self-respect while being mindful of the other person's feelings. This balance is key in creating and sustaining healthy, supportive relationships. Role-playing exercises and group therapy sessions often form part of this learning process, helping individuals practice and refine their communication strategies in a safe environment.

## Integrating DBT with Personal Experience

One of the most powerful aspects of DBT is that it is both a cognitive and experiential therapy. It doesn't simply instruct you on what to do in a given moment—it helps you understand the "why" behind your actions and emotions. In my own journey, DBT has been a transformative tool. I recall moments when I felt utterly overwhelmed by my emotions, convinced that I was destined to repeat destructive patterns. It was through the structured practice of mindfulness and the step-by-step approach to emotion regulation that I began to see my feelings not as an uncontrollable force, but as signals that could guide me toward healthier behaviors.

Journaling became a vital part of this process. By recording my emotions and the situations that triggered them, I was able to identify recurring patterns. Over time, I learned to anticipate certain emotional responses and employ distress tolerance strategies before the situation escalated. This proactive approach was not an immediate fix but a gradual process of learning and adaptation—one that required both self-compassion and perseverance.

## Beyond DBT: Complementary Coping Tools

While DBT is a highly effective framework, it is not the only tool available for managing BPD. Many women find that combining DBT with other therapeutic approaches can enhance their overall well-being.

### Mindfulness-Based Stress Reduction (MBSR)

MBSR is a structured program that teaches mindfulness meditation as a means of reducing stress. Like DBT, it encourages you to be present in the moment and to observe your thoughts and feelings without judgment. Incorporating elements of MBSR can deepen your mindfulness practice, making it easier to apply these skills during times of stress. Techniques learned through MBSR can complement DBT's mindfulness modules, providing additional strategies for grounding yourself.

### Acceptance and Commitment Therapy (ACT)

ACT focuses on accepting your emotions and committing to behaviors that align with your values. It emphasizes the importance of psychological flexibility—the ability to stay in contact with the present moment and to change or persist in behavior that aligns with your long-term goals. ACT's emphasis on values-based living can help you navigate the complexities of BPD by encouraging you to make choices that are in line with your authentic self, even when emotions are running high.

## *Expressive Arts Therapies*

For many, traditional talk therapy may not be enough to fully express the depth of their emotions. Expressive arts therapies, including art, music, and writing therapy, offer alternative outlets for self-expression and healing. These creative approaches can help you process emotions that are difficult to articulate in words, serving as a bridge between your internal experiences and the external world. Many women have found that engaging in creative expression not only alleviates stress but also reinforces their sense of identity and empowerment.

## Practical Exercises to Get Started

To help you integrate these coping tools into your daily life, here are a few exercises that blend the core principles of DBT with complementary techniques:

## *Mindful Breathing Exercise*

1. **Find a Quiet Space:** Sit comfortably in a quiet space where you will not be disturbed.
2. **Focus on Your Breath:** Close your eyes and focus your attention on your breathing. Notice the sensation of air filling your lungs and then slowly leaving your body.
3. **Count Your Breaths:** To anchor your attention, count each breath cycle. If your mind wanders, gently bring your focus back to your breath.
4. **Practice for 10 Minutes:** Aim to practice this mindful breathing exercise for at least 10 minutes a day. This simple practice can help center you during moments of stress.

## Distress Tolerance Toolkit

1. **Create a List:** Make a list of activities or items that help soothe or distract you. This could include listening to calming music, holding a comforting object, or engaging in a brief walk.
2. **Use the "TIP" Skills:** When you're in a state of high distress, try using the TIP skills: change your body temperature (splash cold water on your face), engage in intense exercise, practice paced breathing, or use progressive muscle relaxation.
3. **Reflect on the Outcome:** After using these techniques, journal about how they made you feel and any changes you noticed in your emotional state.

## Emotion Regulation Journal

1. **Daily Log:** Keep a daily journal where you log your emotions, their intensity, and the situations that triggered them.
2. **Identify Patterns:** Over time, look for patterns in your emotional responses. What situations consistently trigger strong emotions? What coping strategies seem to work best?
3. **Set Small Goals:** Based on your observations, set small, achievable goals for managing your emotions. For example, if you notice that a particular stressor consistently leads to overwhelming sadness, plan a strategy to address it using the DBT skills you're learning.

## Interpersonal Role-Playing

1. **Practice Conversations:** Role-play challenging conversations with a trusted friend or therapist. This can help you experiment with different ways of expressing your needs and setting boundaries.
2. **Feedback Loop:** Ask for feedback on your communication style.

What worked well? What might be improved? This exercise not only enhances your interpersonal skills but also builds your confidence in navigating real-life interactions.

## Integrating Skills into Daily Life

One of the challenges many women face when learning new coping skills is applying them consistently in the midst of life's chaos. It is important to remember that progress is rarely linear. Some days, you may find it easier to use mindfulness or emotion regulation techniques, while on other days, distress tolerance skills may be your primary lifeline.

Consistency comes with practice, and the goal is not to eliminate distress entirely but to build a buffer between your emotions and your reactions. Over time, the small, everyday applications of these skills can lead to significant changes in how you respond to stress and interact with others. As you integrate these practices into your daily routine, you may find that what once felt like a series of insurmountable challenges gradually becomes a series of manageable moments—and each moment is an opportunity for growth.

## Personal Reflections on the Journey

Learning DBT and related coping tools has been transformative in my journey toward managing BPD. There were moments when I felt completely overwhelmed by my emotional landscape, as if I were drowning in a sea of intensity. DBT provided me with the tools to not only recognize the waves but to ride them. I began to understand that my emotional responses, while sometimes overwhelming, were not insurmountable. Instead, they were signals—a call for me to pause, reflect, and choose a response that honored both my pain and my strength.

Through years of practice, I've seen firsthand how the mindful awareness of my emotions can lead to better decision-making and improved relationships. The skills of distress tolerance helped me navigate crises without resorting to behaviors that I later regretted. And as I honed my ability to regulate my emotions and communicate more effectively, I began to see a gradual shift in my interactions with others— moving from a cycle of conflict to a more balanced, authentic way of relating.

## The Road Ahead

In embracing DBT and other coping tools, you are taking an important step toward reclaiming your emotional life. This journey is not about perfection—it is about progress, one small step at a time. The techniques you learn here are meant to serve as a foundation upon which you can build a more resilient, empowered self. There will be setbacks and challenges along the way, but with each setback comes an opportunity to learn, to adapt, and to grow stronger.

As you continue through this book, remember that the skills you develop here are lifelong companions. They are not a cure-all, but they can help transform moments of crisis into opportunities for growth. The process of learning, practicing, and integrating these tools is a journey in itself—one that requires patience, perseverance, and above all, self-compassion.

This chapter has provided an introduction to DBT and other coping tools that have proven effective in managing the complexities of BPD. From the foundational practices of mindfulness and emotion regulation to the practical strategies of distress tolerance and interpersonal effectiveness, each tool is designed to help you navigate the emotional storms and interpersonal challenges that come with living a life marked by intensity.

By incorporating these skills into your daily life—through exercises, journaling, and even role-playing—you lay the groundwork for a more balanced, resilient self. The journey toward emotional regulation is ongoing, and every practice session, every moment of mindfulness, is a step toward reclaiming your narrative.

As you move forward, allow yourself the space to learn, adapt, and evolve. Embrace the small victories and be gentle with yourself in moments of struggle. Remember that every effort you make is an affirmation of your strength and a commitment to living a life that honors both your vulnerabilities and your extraordinary capacity for growth.

In the chapters ahead, we will continue to build on these foundational skills, exploring further strategies to create lasting change and empower you to live beyond the constraints of BPD. Until then, may the insights and practices of DBT and related coping tools serve as a steady guide on your journey toward a more harmonious, fulfilled life.

# 6

# Deep Dive into Mindfulness and Emotional Regulation

Mindfulness and emotional regulation stand at the core of effective coping strategies for Borderline Personality Disorder (BPD). For many women with BPD, intense emotions often feel uncontrollable and overwhelming. In this chapter, we take a deep dive into the practices of mindfulness and emotional regulation—two essential tools that work hand-in-hand to transform the way you experience and manage your emotions. By exploring their theoretical foundations, practical applications, and personal reflections, this chapter offers a comprehensive guide to harnessing these techniques for a more balanced and empowered life.

# Understanding Mindfulness: The Art of Present-Moment Awareness

At its simplest, mindfulness is the practice of fully attending to the present moment without judgment. It is an invitation to step out of the habitual cycle of rumination and anxiety and to observe your thoughts, feelings, and sensations as they arise. For women living with BPD, whose emotional responses can often feel intense and unpredictable, mindfulness provides a gentle space to pause and gain perspective.

## The Origins and Evolution of Mindfulness

Mindfulness has deep roots in ancient meditation practices, yet its modern adaptation—especially within Dialectical Behavior Therapy (DBT)—has made it accessible for managing emotional distress. In DBT, mindfulness is not about escaping reality; rather, it is about accepting it fully. It encourages you to acknowledge both pleasant and unpleasant experiences without clinging to them or pushing them away.

Numerous studies have highlighted the benefits of mindfulness in reducing stress and improving emotional balance. For example, mindfulness practices have been shown to decrease activity in the brain's stress centers while increasing connectivity in areas responsible for emotional regulation. These neurological shifts underscore the powerful impact that consistent mindfulness practice can have on our overall mental well-being.

## Practical Mindfulness Techniques

One of the simplest ways to incorporate mindfulness into your daily life is through mindful breathing exercises. Here is a step-by-step guide to get started:

1. **Find a Quiet Place:** Sit comfortably in a quiet space. Close your eyes and allow your body to relax.
2. **Focus on Your Breath:** Bring your attention to the sensation of breathing. Notice the coolness of the air as you inhale and the warmth as you exhale.
3. **Observe Without Judgment:** As thoughts arise, simply acknowledge them without engaging. Imagine them as clouds drifting across a sky.
4. **Return to the Breath:** Gently bring your attention back to your breath each time you notice your mind wandering.
5. **Practice Consistently:** Start with 5–10 minutes each day, gradually increasing the duration as you feel more comfortable.

Mindful walking or body scans are also excellent practices. These techniques allow you to tune into your physical sensations, making it easier to identify where you might be holding tension or stress. Over time, these practices can help you notice early signs of emotional escalation, giving you the opportunity to intervene before a full-blown crisis occurs.

## Personal Reflections on Mindfulness

In my own journey, I found that mindfulness was not an instant fix but a gradual process of learning and acceptance. Initially, sitting still with my thoughts was challenging—my mind would race with worries and memories. However, as I practiced daily, I began to notice subtle shifts. Moments of anxiety became more manageable, and I started to appreciate the clarity that came with being fully present. Mindfulness transformed my relationship with my emotions, helping me see them as temporary states rather than overwhelming forces.

## Emotional Regulation: Balancing the Inner Landscape

While mindfulness lays the groundwork for awareness, emotional regulation provides the tools to manage and balance the spectrum of feelings that come with BPD. Emotional regulation is the process by which you learn to understand, label, and modify your emotional responses. It involves not only reducing the intensity of negative emotions but also fostering the capacity to experience positive emotions more fully.

### *What is Emotional Regulation?*

Emotional regulation refers to the ability to manage one's emotional responses in a way that is adaptive and aligned with personal goals. For many women with BPD, emotions can feel like tidal waves—sudden, overwhelming, and all-consuming. Emotional regulation skills empower you to ride these waves rather than be swept away by them.

These skills can be broken down into several key components:

- **Identifying Emotions:** The first step is learning to accurately label your emotions. Keeping an emotion diary can be a useful tool here.
- **Understanding Triggers:** Recognizing the situations or thoughts that spark intense emotions is crucial for preventing emotional spirals.
- **Developing Coping Strategies:** Once you know your triggers, you can apply specific strategies—such as deep breathing, visualization, or engaging in a distracting activity—to modulate your emotional intensity.
- **Reflecting and Reframing:** After an emotional episode, reflecting on what happened and how you managed it can build resilience and inform future strategies.

## *Techniques for Effective Emotional Regulation*

Here are several techniques to help you cultivate better emotional regulation:

1. **Emotion Journaling:** Keep a daily log of your emotions. Write down what you feel, the intensity of those emotions, and any triggers or events that seem connected. Over time, patterns will emerge, helping you anticipate and prepare for emotional shifts.
2. **Cognitive Reappraisal:** This is the practice of reinterpreting a situation in a way that alters its emotional impact. For example, if you feel rejected because a friend canceled plans, try to view it as an opportunity for self-care rather than a personal failure.
3. **Progressive Muscle Relaxation:** Tension in the body can amplify emotional distress. This technique involves slowly tensing and then relaxing different muscle groups to promote physical and emotional calmness.
4. **Visualization:** Imagine a safe, peaceful place or visualize your emotions as a river, flowing and changing over time. This mental imagery can provide a sense of distance and control over your feelings.

## *Integrating Mindfulness and Emotional Regulation*

The power of these practices lies in their integration. When you combine mindfulness with emotional regulation, you create a dynamic framework for handling emotions. Mindfulness helps you become aware of your feelings in real-time, while emotional regulation provides the methods to manage them constructively.

For instance, if you notice a surge of anger during a conflict, mindfulness allows you to observe the sensation without immediately reacting. Once you're aware, you can then apply an emotional regulation strategy—perhaps deep breathing or cognitive reappraisal—to defuse the intensity and approach the situation more calmly. Over time, this combined practice can help you break free from reactive cycles and build more balanced emotional responses.

## Real-Life Applications and Challenges

Applying mindfulness and emotional regulation in the heat of the moment can be challenging. There will be times when, despite your best efforts, emotions feel overwhelming. This is a natural part of the process, and setbacks are not failures—they are opportunities for learning and growth.

One effective approach is to plan ahead for emotionally charged situations. For example, if you know that certain social settings trigger anxiety or anger, prepare by practicing mindfulness exercises beforehand. Keep a set of distress tolerance tools handy, and remind yourself that it's okay to take a break or excuse yourself if you need to regroup.

Another common challenge is the tendency to revert to old habits during periods of high stress. In these moments, self-compassion is key. Acknowledge that change is gradual and that every attempt to use these skills, even if imperfect, contributes to long-term progress. Remember that even a few moments of mindful awareness or a brief pause to regulate your emotions are steps in the right direction.

## Case Example: Navigating a Conflict

Consider a scenario where a heated conversation with a loved one escalates into a potential conflict. In the past, such moments might have led to impulsive reactions, further damaging the relationship. With a foundation in mindfulness, you might first notice your body tensing and your heart rate increasing. A quick mindful breathing exercise—pausing to focus solely on your breath—can create the space needed to choose a more measured response. Next, applying emotional regulation strategies like cognitive reappraisal, you might remind yourself that the conflict does not define your relationship, but rather is an opportunity to understand each other better. By using these techniques together, you may navigate the situation with greater clarity and less emotional turmoil, ultimately fostering healthier communication.

## The Role of Practice and Patience

Mastering mindfulness and emotional regulation is not an overnight process. It requires consistent practice and a willingness to accept imperfection. There will be days when mindfulness feels elusive or when emotions seem too powerful to control. During these times, revisit your practices with kindness. Celebrate the small victories—a few minutes of focused breathing, a moment of clear self-awareness, or a successful use of a regulation strategy during a stressful moment.

One practical tip is to set aside a dedicated time each day for these practices. Whether it's a morning meditation session or a quiet moment before bed, creating a routine helps embed these skills into your daily life. Over time, these practices will become more natural, enabling you to access them even during moments of crisis.

## Reflections on the Journey

In my own journey with BPD, integrating mindfulness and emotional regulation has been transformative. There were periods when emotions felt like uncontrollable storms, but the gradual accumulation of mindful moments and regulatory techniques allowed me to build an inner sanctuary—a space where I could observe and manage my feelings rather than be overwhelmed by them. I learned that it wasn't about eliminating emotions, but about understanding their transient nature and recognizing that each emotional surge was an invitation to respond rather than react.

This journey is deeply personal and unique. While the techniques outlined here have been widely beneficial, it's important to adapt them to your own needs and experiences. Experiment with different exercises, reflect on what resonates with you, and modify practices to fit your personal rhythm. Your path to emotional balance is as individual as you are.

## Moving Forward

As we close this chapter, consider the practices of mindfulness and emotional regulation as foundational pillars on your journey toward emotional resilience. Each moment spent in mindful reflection, every instance of successfully navigating a challenging emotion, contributes to building a more stable and empowered self. The techniques you learn here will not only help manage the intensity of BPD but will also enrich your overall experience of life—allowing you to savor moments of joy, navigate periods of sorrow, and ultimately cultivate a deeper understanding of who you are.

In the chapters to come, we will build on these skills, exploring ways to further integrate them into your interpersonal relationships and daily routines. The journey is ongoing, filled with learning, adaptation, and profound growth. Embrace each step with compassion and curiosity, knowing that every practice session brings you closer to the balanced, resilient life you deserve.

In conclusion, mindfulness and emotional regulation are not merely abstract concepts—they are practical, transformative tools that can reshape your relationship with your emotions. By anchoring yourself in the present moment and learning to modulate your emotional responses, you gain the power to transform overwhelming feelings into manageable, even insightful, experiences. With practice and patience, these skills will become a trusted part of your daily life, supporting you through challenges and enriching your moments of calm.

May the practices in this chapter serve as a beacon on your journey— reminding you that even in the midst of emotional intensity, there is always an opportunity to pause, reflect, and choose a path of balance and self-compassion.

# 7

# Building and Maintaining Healthy Relationships

Relationships are both a source of profound fulfillment and a challenge for many women living with BPD. The emotional intensity that characterizes our internal worlds can create a turbulent dynamic with loved ones—friends, family, partners, and even colleagues. In this chapter, we explore the art and science of building and maintaining healthy relationships. Drawing from personal reflections, clinical insights, and practical exercises from therapies like Dialectical Behavior Therapy (DBT), we will navigate the terrain of connection, setting boundaries, and fostering trust.

## The Importance of Connection

Human connection is at the core of our emotional well-being. From the moment we are born, relationships shape our self-concept and help us form our identity. For many women with BPD, however, early experiences of inconsistent care or emotionally charged environments can lead to a deep-seated fear of abandonment and difficulty trusting others. These challenges may manifest as intense attachments or sudden withdrawals, making relationships feel like a constant tightrope walk.

In my own journey, I often felt caught between an overwhelming need for closeness and the equally powerful impulse to retreat when I sensed rejection or criticism. Over time, I learned that healthy relationships require both vulnerability and structure—a balance that allows us to be authentic while feeling secure.

## Understanding Interpersonal Effectiveness

Interpersonal effectiveness is a cornerstone of DBT and an essential skill for managing relationships. It involves learning to communicate your needs, assert boundaries, and negotiate conflicts without sacrificing your self-respect or the connection you share with others. This skill set is particularly vital for women with BPD, who may struggle with extreme reactions during interpersonal conflicts.

## Core Components of Interpersonal Effectiveness

1. **Assertiveness:** This means expressing your thoughts, feelings, and needs directly and respectfully. Assertiveness is not about being aggressive; it's about stating your truth clearly. Role-playing exercises, as suggested in DBT modules, can be incredibly useful for practicing this skill.
2. **Active Listening:** Healthy communication is a two-way street. Active listening involves fully focusing on the speaker, acknowledging their perspective, and validating their feelings. This practice helps to build trust and fosters mutual understanding.
3. **Boundary Setting:** Boundaries are the invisible lines that protect your emotional space. Learning to set and maintain clear boundaries is crucial, especially if past experiences have left you feeling overwhelmed or taken advantage of. A boundary might be

as simple as explaining to a friend when you need some alone time to recharge.

4. **Conflict Resolution:** Disagreements are inevitable in any relationship. The key is to manage conflicts constructively. Techniques such as taking a time-out, using "I" statements to express your feelings, and brainstorming mutually acceptable solutions are all part of effective conflict resolution.

## Recognizing Patterns and Triggers in Relationships

A vital step in improving relationships is recognizing the patterns that might be sabotaging them. Many women with BPD experience a recurring cycle: moments of intense closeness followed by dramatic distancing. This "push-pull" dynamic often stems from an underlying fear of abandonment and can be exacerbated by misinterpretations of others' actions.

### Self-Reflection and Journaling

One powerful tool for understanding these patterns is journaling. Keeping a relationship journal allows you to record interactions, note your emotional responses, and identify triggers that lead to conflict. Over time, you might notice that certain topics or situations consistently provoke a strong reaction. For instance, criticism—even when constructive—might trigger a deep-seated fear of rejection, leading you to withdraw or lash out.

In my own practice, I found that reflecting on these moments with a neutral, non-judgmental lens helped me develop greater insight into my emotional patterns. With this awareness, I could then apply DBT skills, such as mindfulness and distress tolerance, to prevent a minor disagreement from escalating into a full-blown crisis.

# Practical Strategies for Building Healthier Relationships

Transforming your approach to relationships involves a blend of self-awareness, effective communication, and consistent practice. Below are several strategies designed to help you cultivate and sustain healthier relationships:

## 1. Establishing Clear Communication

Clear, honest communication is the foundation of every strong relationship. Here are a few steps to enhance your communication skills:

- **Use "I" Statements:** Instead of saying, "You never listen to me," try, "I feel unheard when I'm interrupted." This approach reduces defensiveness and centers the conversation on your feelings.
- **Clarify Your Needs:** Before entering a conversation, take a moment to pinpoint what you need from the interaction. Are you looking for advice, validation, or simply to be heard?
- **Practice Active Listening:** Encourage a dialogue by reflecting back what the other person says. This practice not only confirms that you understand their perspective but also fosters a sense of mutual respect.

## 2. Setting and Respecting Boundaries

Boundaries are crucial for maintaining a sense of self within relationships. Here are some steps to create healthy boundaries:

- **Identify Your Limits:** Reflect on situations where you feel drained, overwhelmed, or disrespected. Write down what behaviors are acceptable and what aren't.

- **Communicate Clearly:** Once you know your limits, articulate them to your loved ones. For example, "I need some quiet time after work to decompress. Can we talk after 8 PM?"
- **Enforce Your Boundaries:** Consistency is key. If your boundaries are crossed, gently but firmly remind the other person of your limits. Over time, both you and those around you will come to respect these boundaries.

## 3. Building a Support Network

No one should have to navigate the complexities of BPD alone. Building a supportive network can provide the emotional sustenance needed during challenging times. Here are ways to cultivate your support system:

- **Join Support Groups:** Look for local or online groups where women with BPD share their experiences. These communities offer validation, practical advice, and a sense of belonging.
- **Lean on Trusted Friends:** Identify individuals who have demonstrated empathy, reliability, and understanding in your past. Reach out to them when you're struggling, and be open about your needs.
- **Seek Professional Guidance:** A therapist, particularly one trained in DBT, can offer invaluable tools and strategies for managing relationship dynamics. Regular therapy sessions can help reinforce the skills you're learning and provide a safe space to process difficult interactions.

## 4. Conflict Resolution Techniques

Even in the healthiest relationships, conflicts arise. How you navigate these moments can significantly impact the longevity and quality of your connections.

- **Pause and Reflect:** When emotions run high, give yourself permission to take a break. This pause can prevent impulsive reactions and provide space for rational thinking.
- **Use Problem-Solving Skills:** Instead of focusing on what went wrong, shift the conversation toward solutions. Ask questions like, "How can we handle this differently next time?"
- **Seek Compromise:** Recognize that both parties may need to adjust. A willingness to compromise is often the key to resolving conflicts in a way that feels respectful and mutually beneficial.

## Personal Reflections on Transformative Relationships

The journey to healthier relationships is deeply personal. I remember a time when even minor disagreements would spiral into intense conflicts. I would alternate between clinging desperately to the person and pushing them away in an attempt to protect myself from potential hurt. Through therapy and the consistent application of DBT skills, I began to see that the intensity of my reactions was a signal—a call for me to pause, reflect, and re-engage with a more balanced approach.

One significant breakthrough came when I learned to recognize the early signs of a conflict brewing. By paying attention to physical cues, such as a tightness in my chest or a racing heartbeat, I was able to pause and use mindfulness to ground myself. This practice allowed me to approach the conversation with greater clarity and less reactivity, ultimately fostering a deeper, more empathetic dialogue. Over time, my relationships began to transform. I noticed that by asserting my needs calmly and respectfully, I not only reduced the frequency of conflicts but also built a stronger, more authentic connection with those around me.

## Challenges and Setbacks

Despite progress, setbacks are an inevitable part of any journey toward healthier relationships. There may be moments when old patterns resurface, when a feeling of abandonment or rejection seems overwhelming, and you find yourself slipping back into familiar, unhelpful behaviors. These setbacks are not failures—they are opportunities for learning and growth.

When setbacks occur, it is essential to practice self-compassion. Acknowledge the difficulty of the situation without judgment. Reflect on what triggered the reaction and consider which DBT skills might have helped in that moment. Over time, this reflective practice can turn setbacks into stepping stones toward even greater emotional resilience.

## Exercises to Enhance Interpersonal Skills

To further support your journey toward building healthier relationships, here are some practical exercises that blend the principles of DBT with everyday scenarios:

### Role-Playing Difficult Conversations

1. **Choose a Scenario:** Identify a common situation that often leads to conflict—perhaps a disagreement over plans or a miscommunication about expectations.
2. **Partner Up:** Find a trusted friend or family member who is willing to participate in a role-playing exercise.
3. **Practice Assertive Communication:** Take turns acting out the conversation, focusing on using "I" statements, active listening, and clear boundary-setting.
4. **Reflect:** After the exercise, discuss what felt effective and what

could be improved. This feedback loop can provide insights and build confidence in real-world situations.

## Journaling Relationship Patterns

1. **Daily Reflection:** Keep a dedicated journal for relationship interactions. Note what went well and what challenges arose.
2. **Identify Patterns:** Over a few weeks, review your entries to see if any recurring themes or triggers emerge.
3. **Set Goals:** Based on your observations, set specific, achievable goals—for example, practicing a new boundary or using assertive communication during a conflict.

## Mindfulness in Relationships

1. **Pre-Conversation Mindfulness:** Before entering a potentially challenging interaction, take a few minutes to practice mindful breathing or a brief meditation. This can help center your emotions and prepare you to respond rather than react.
2. **Post-Conversation Reflection:** After a conversation, take time to reflect on how you felt and whether you were able to use your DBT skills effectively. Over time, this can reinforce positive behaviors and highlight areas for further growth.

## Cultivating Self-Awareness and Empathy

Building and maintaining healthy relationships also requires a continuous commitment to self-awareness and empathy—both for yourself and for those around you. By regularly engaging in self-reflection, you can identify the ways in which your emotional patterns influence your interactions. This awareness is the first step toward change.

Empathy plays a dual role in relationships: it allows you to connect with others on a deeper level and also helps you understand your own emotional landscape. When you practice empathy toward yourself, you create a compassionate internal environment where mistakes become opportunities for learning rather than sources of shame.

## Looking to the Future

As you continue to develop your interpersonal skills, remember that relationships are living, evolving entities. They require continuous care, attention, and mutual effort. Every positive interaction builds a foundation of trust and respect that can weather even the most challenging storms. The tools and strategies discussed in this chapter are not meant to eliminate conflict altogether but to transform the way you experience and resolve it.

In the chapters that follow, we will further explore how to reclaim and redefine your personal identity and narrative in the context of living with BPD. Healthy relationships are both a mirror and a support system— they reflect back your growth and provide the strength to move forward, even when the path is difficult.

## Final Thoughts

The journey to building and maintaining healthy relationships is both challenging and deeply rewarding. By integrating the principles of interpersonal effectiveness with mindful self-reflection, you can forge connections that honor your authentic self while fostering growth and mutual respect. Whether you are mending strained relationships or forging new bonds, remember that each interaction is an opportunity to practice self-compassion, assertiveness, and empathy.

As you reflect on the strategies discussed in this chapter, consider them not as a strict set of rules, but as flexible tools designed to empower you. With time, patience, and consistent practice, you can create relationships that nurture your well-being and celebrate the resilience and depth of your emotional world.

May the insights and exercises offered here serve as a guide as you navigate the complexities of connection. Embrace the journey with an open heart and know that each step you take—each honest conversation, every boundary set with clarity—brings you closer to the balanced, fulfilling relationships you deserve.

# 8

# Rediscovering and Embracing Your Identity

One of the most transformative parts of the journey with Borderline Personality Disorder (BPD) is the process of rediscovering and embracing your identity. For many women, years of internalizing societal expectations, grappling with early traumas, and living with the stigma of BPD can obscure a true sense of self. This chapter is an invitation to explore who you are beyond the diagnosis—a multifaceted individual with strengths, passions, and unique qualities that define your essence. In these pages, we will examine how to peel away the layers of imposed identity, reclaim your personal narrative, and embrace a more authentic, empowered self.

## The Struggle to Define the "Self"

For years, I felt that my identity was tangled up in labels: "unstable," "difficult," "emotionally volatile." The clinical language surrounding BPD often reduced my experiences to a set of symptoms, leaving little room for the richness of my personality. In our culture, where women are frequently expected to fit into predetermined roles—nurturer, caregiver, peacemaker—the intense emotions and inner conflicts that come with

BPD were seen as deviations rather than expressions of a vibrant inner life.

Many women with BPD share this experience. Early relationships and social conditioning can lead us to suppress parts of ourselves to be accepted. Over time, the fear of abandonment or judgment can force us into roles that feel safe but do not truly represent who we are. This conflict between the "public" self and the "true" self can leave a lasting impression of disconnection. Yet, it is possible—and deeply liberating—to dismantle these layers and reclaim your unique identity.

## The Journey Toward Self-Discovery

Self-discovery is not a destination; it is an ongoing process of exploration and acceptance. It involves looking inward with honest curiosity, reflecting on your experiences, and acknowledging the parts of you that may have been hidden or denied. Here are several steps that can help guide you on this journey:

### 1. Reflecting on Your Past

Our early experiences leave imprints on who we become. Reflecting on your past is essential—not to dwell on pain, but to understand the forces that shaped your identity. Consider journaling about:

- **Key Life Events:** Write about moments that have defined you. How have these events contributed to your strengths as well as your vulnerabilities?
- **Family Narratives:** Explore the roles you were assigned in your family. Did you become the "sensitive one," the "caretaker," or perhaps the "troubled" child? Understanding these roles can help you decide which parts of that narrative you want to keep and which

you wish to redefine.

- **Cultural Influences:** Think about the societal expectations that were placed on you as a woman. How did these influence your behaviors, choices, and sense of self?

By reflecting on these aspects, you can begin to see the layers that have accumulated over time and decide which ones serve you—and which ones no longer do.

## 2. Identifying Your Values and Passions

Rediscovering your identity means reconnecting with the parts of you that feel authentic and fulfilling. Ask yourself:

- **What truly matters?** Identify your core values—honesty, creativity, compassion, resilience—and consider how they align with your daily life.
- **What activities make you feel alive?** Engage in hobbies, creative pursuits, or social causes that resonate with your inner self. Whether it's writing, painting, dancing, or volunteering, these passions can reveal aspects of your identity that have long been suppressed.
- **What kind of relationships nourish you?** Reflect on the connections that have helped you feel seen and understood. Relationships that encourage you to be your true self are essential in fostering a positive self-image.

When you align your life with your values and passions, you begin to create a life narrative that is uniquely yours—one that is not defined solely by a diagnosis but enriched by your talents, interests, and dreams.

## 3. Challenging Internalized Narratives

One of the most powerful steps in embracing your identity is challenging the negative beliefs that have been ingrained in you over the years. Many women with BPD internalize messages of inadequacy, often hearing themselves described as "too much" or "not enough." These internalized narratives can distort self-perception and limit personal growth.

- **Practice Self-Compassion:** Treat yourself with the same kindness and understanding that you would offer a dear friend. Recognize that mistakes and emotional fluctuations are part of being human, not evidence of failure.
- **Cognitive Restructuring:** When you catch yourself thinking, "I'm broken" or "I can't change," pause and reframe these thoughts. Replace them with affirmations like, "I am a work in progress, and I have unique strengths," or "My emotions are a part of me, not a definition of my worth."
- **Seek Evidence of Your Strengths:** Create a list of your accomplishments, however small, and the qualities that make you who you are. Reflect on moments when you overcame challenges or acted in alignment with your values.

By actively questioning and reframing these narratives, you create space for a more balanced, compassionate view of yourself.

## Embracing Authenticity Through Creative Expression

Creative expression is a powerful way to tap into and share your inner self. Whether you enjoy writing, art, music, or any other form of creative outlet, these practices can serve as both a mirror and a canvas for your identity.

## Art as a Reflection of Self

For many women, art becomes a language through which emotions can be expressed without words. Painting or drawing can help externalize feelings that are otherwise difficult to articulate. When you engage in creative activities, you invite your inner world to take form—allowing you to see and appreciate the beauty and complexity within you.

## Journaling as a Tool for Self-Exploration

Journaling remains one of the most effective tools for rediscovering your identity. Set aside time daily or weekly to reflect on your thoughts and experiences. Use prompts such as:

- "What do I love about myself today?"
- "What emotions have surfaced, and what might they be telling me about my needs?"
- "What dreams or aspirations have I pushed aside, and how can I bring them back into focus?"

Over time, your journal will become a personal narrative—a testament to your evolving identity and the journey toward embracing your authentic self.

## The Therapeutic Value of Storytelling

Sharing your story can be a liberating and validating experience. Whether through memoir, support groups, or online communities, storytelling allows you to connect with others who may have faced similar challenges. It also serves as a reminder that your experiences have shaped you in unique ways that can inspire and empower both yourself and those around you.

## Cultivating a Growth Mindset

Embracing your identity involves adopting a growth mindset—a belief that you can continue to evolve and improve throughout your life. This perspective encourages you to view challenges as opportunities for growth rather than as insurmountable obstacles.

- **Celebrate Small Victories:** Each step you take toward understanding and embracing your true self is a victory. Whether it's speaking up in a challenging conversation or resisting old patterns, recognize and celebrate your progress.
- **Be Open to Change:** Understand that your identity is not fixed; it is fluid and dynamic. Allow yourself the flexibility to grow, change, and explore new aspects of who you are.
- **Learn from Setbacks:** When you encounter setbacks, reflect on them without judgment. Ask yourself what these experiences teach you and how they can inform your journey forward.

By nurturing a growth mindset, you empower yourself to view every experience—whether positive or challenging—as a part of your evolving narrative.

## Integrating Therapy and Self-Reflection

Professional therapy can provide invaluable support as you navigate the complexities of identity formation. Therapeutic approaches such as Dialectical Behavior Therapy (DBT) and psychodynamic therapy offer frameworks for understanding how past experiences and emotional patterns have shaped your identity.

- **DBT and Identity:** In DBT, mindfulness and emotional regulation skills can help you observe your internal states without judgment, creating space for self-reflection. This process allows you to differentiate between emotions triggered by past experiences and those that reflect your authentic self.
- **Exploring Self with a Therapist:** A therapist can guide you in unpacking the layers of your identity, helping you understand how societal expectations and personal history have influenced your self-perception. Through reflective dialogue and targeted exercises, you can begin to separate your true desires and values from the imposed narratives of others.
- **Group Therapy and Peer Support:** Engaging in group therapy or support groups can also reinforce your sense of self. Hearing others' stories and sharing your own can normalize the struggles of identity formation, reminding you that you are not alone in this journey.

Therapy, when combined with personal reflection and creative expression, offers a holistic approach to rediscovering and embracing your identity.

## Crafting a New Narrative

As you sift through the layers of your past and reconnect with your true self, you are essentially crafting a new narrative—one that is honest, empowering, and uniquely yours. This new narrative does not erase the challenges of living with BPD; rather, it integrates them into a broader story of resilience, growth, and transformation.

- **Rewriting Your Story:** Begin by identifying the chapters of your life that you no longer wish to define you. Then, consciously write new chapters that highlight your strengths, aspirations, and moments of triumph. This exercise can be as creative as writing a memoir, creating a vision board, or even composing a song that captures your journey.
- **Affirmations and Positive Self-Talk:** Develop affirmations that resonate with your redefined identity. Phrases like "I am more than my diagnosis" or "My emotions are a part of me, and they empower me" can serve as daily reminders of your inherent worth.
- **Living Authentically:** The ultimate goal of redefining your identity is to live in a way that feels true to who you are. This may mean making changes in your relationships, career, or lifestyle that align with your values and passions. Authentic living is a continuous process of making choices that honor your true self, even when external pressures try to steer you back into old patterns.

## Embracing Your Unique Strengths

Throughout this journey, it's important to acknowledge and celebrate the unique strengths that come with living a life marked by intensity and sensitivity. Many women with BPD have a profound capacity for empathy, creativity, and deep connection—qualities that are invaluable in a world that often values conformity over individuality.

- **Empathy as a Gift:** Your ability to feel deeply can be a tremendous asset. It allows you to connect with others in meaningful ways and to offer insights that only someone who has experienced intense emotions can provide.
- **Creativity Born of Intensity:** The very traits that make your emotions overwhelming can also fuel creative expression. Many artists,

writers, and innovators have harnessed their emotional depth to create works that resonate on a profound level.

- **Resilience Through Struggle:** Every challenge you have overcome contributes to your inner strength. The very process of navigating life with BPD builds resilience—a strength that can inspire others and fortify you in times of hardship.

## Final Reflections on Identity

Rediscovering and embracing your identity is a lifelong journey that requires courage, reflection, and self-compassion. It means daring to peel away the layers of externally imposed labels and reconnecting with the essence of who you are. This process may be challenging, and there may be moments of uncertainty or discomfort as old narratives are dismantled. Yet, every step you take toward understanding your true self is a testament to your resilience and capacity for growth.

In embracing your identity, you learn to see your experiences not as burdens but as integral parts of a rich, evolving narrative. Your journey is not defined solely by the struggles of BPD but by the unique qualities, passions, and strengths that make you who you are. As you move forward, remember that you have the power to rewrite your story— one that celebrates both the challenges you have overcome and the bright possibilities that lie ahead.

May this chapter serve as both a guide and an inspiration as you continue your journey of self-discovery. Embrace the process with openness and curiosity, and trust that every reflection, every creative expression, and every act of self-compassion is a step toward a more authentic, empowered you.

In the chapters that follow, we will continue to build on these themes— exploring ways to further integrate your rediscovered identity into every aspect of your life. For now, take a moment to honor the progress you have made. Recognize that your identity is not fixed or limited by a diagnosis; it is as expansive and dynamic as the life you are choosing to create.

By reclaiming your identity, you are not only embracing yourself more fully—you are also setting an example for others who may be struggling with similar challenges. Your journey toward self-discovery has the power to inspire, uplift, and transform both your life and the lives of those around you. Embrace your unique story, and know that every step you take is a step toward a future that honors the true you.

May the insights and practices shared in this chapter empower you to live more authentically, boldly, and compassionately. Embrace the beautiful complexity of your identity, celebrate your strengths, and allow yourself the freedom to be exactly who you are—without apology, without reservation, and with a deep, unwavering sense of self-worth.

# 9

# Healing Through Narrative – The Power of Personal Stories

Our lives are woven from the stories we tell ourselves and share with others. For women living with Borderline Personality Disorder (BPD), personal narratives are not only a record of struggle but also a powerful instrument for healing and transformation. In this chapter, we explore how storytelling—whether through writing, art, or conversation—can be a pathway to reclaiming your voice, reinterpreting your past, and forging a future grounded in hope and resilience.

## The Therapeutic Value of Storytelling

Throughout history, storytelling has been central to human connection and healing. When we share our experiences, we give voice to emotions that might otherwise remain locked inside us. For many women with BPD, whose lives are often marked by intense emotional experiences and fragmented narratives, crafting a cohesive story can provide a sense of coherence and meaning.

## The Science Behind Narrative Therapy

Research in narrative psychology suggests that how we frame our experiences influences both our emotional well-being and our behavior. By actively re-authoring our personal narratives, we can challenge destructive self-beliefs and open up new possibilities for growth. Studies indicate that writing about traumatic events, for example, can help reduce stress and improve mental health outcomes. Narrative therapy leverages this power, helping individuals transform their life stories from ones defined by pain into ones that highlight strength, resilience, and recovery.

## Influential Works on Narrative and Healing

Many books have explored the intersection of narrative and healing. In *The Body Keeps the Score* by Bessel van der Kolk, the author shows how trauma is stored in the body and how recounting one's story can facilitate recovery. Similarly, *Man's Search for Meaning* by Viktor Frankl underscores the importance of finding purpose and meaning even amidst suffering. These works remind us that our personal narratives are not static but can be reshaped into powerful tools for reclaiming our identities.

## Unpacking Your Story: A Journey of Self-Discovery

Healing through narrative begins with a willingness to explore the many layers of your story. This journey of self-discovery involves looking deeply at your past experiences, the emotions they evoke, and the ways they have shaped your identity. The process is not about reliving pain but about understanding and integrating your experiences into a broader, more empowering narrative.

## Reflective Writing and Journaling

One of the most accessible ways to begin this journey is through journaling. A dedicated journal can serve as a safe space where you record your thoughts, feelings, and memories without judgment. Consider using prompts such as:

- "What are some pivotal moments in my life, and what did I learn from them?"
- "How have my experiences shaped who I am today, both the challenges and the strengths?"
- "What aspects of my story do I want to honor and preserve?"

By consistently writing about your experiences, you gradually create a coherent narrative that acknowledges both your pain and your progress. Over time, you may discover recurring themes or patterns that offer insights into your emotional life. Journaling not only helps organize your thoughts but also validates your experiences, reinforcing that every chapter of your life—no matter how painful—has contributed to your growth.

## Creative Expression: Art, Music, and Beyond

While words are a powerful medium, creative expression can also serve as a potent vehicle for healing. Many women with BPD find that art, music, or dance provides an alternative way to express emotions that are difficult to articulate verbally. Engaging in creative activities allows you to explore your inner landscape in a non-linear, intuitive way. Painting or drawing, for example, might help you externalize feelings of chaos and intensity, gradually transforming them into visual symbols of resilience and hope.

Consider setting aside time each week for a creative project—whether it's sketching your emotions, composing a piece of music, or even creating a scrapbook of your favorite memories. These projects not only foster self-expression but also create tangible records of your journey, which you can revisit during times of difficulty to remind yourself of how far you've come.

## Sharing Your Story: Finding Your Voice

The act of sharing your story—whether through conversation, group therapy, or public writing—can be incredibly empowering. When you share your narrative, you challenge the stigma that often surrounds BPD and remind others that healing is possible. This process can begin in small, intimate settings. For instance, you might start by sharing your experiences with a trusted friend, a supportive family member, or a mental health professional.

In support groups or online communities dedicated to mental health, you may discover that your story resonates with others. The act of telling your story in these spaces can build a sense of belonging and validation. Hearing others' narratives, too, can offer new perspectives and inspire hope, reminding you that you are not alone in your journey. As Susanna Kaysen's *Girl, Interrupted* and similar memoirs illustrate, personal narratives can spark conversations that challenge societal misconceptions and foster deeper understanding.

## Rewriting Your Narrative: Tools and Techniques

Once you have gathered the raw materials of your story through reflection and creative expression, the next step is to actively rewrite your narrative. This process involves reframing negative experiences and highlighting the strengths and insights that have emerged from them.

## Cognitive Restructuring Through Writing

Cognitive restructuring is a therapeutic technique that involves identifying and challenging negative thought patterns. In the context of
narrative healing, it means re-examining the way you interpret your
past. Ask yourself:

- How might I view this challenging experience as a source of strength
  or learning?
- What positive qualities did I develop as a result of overcoming this
  adversity?
- In what ways have these experiences prepared me to face future
  challenges with resilience?

By answering these questions in writing, you can start to replace
narratives of victimhood with stories of empowerment. This isn't about
diminishing the pain you experienced, but rather about acknowledging
that within that pain lies the potential for growth and transformation.

## Creating a Life Story Outline

Another effective technique is to create an outline of your life story,
dividing it into distinct chapters. Consider structuring your narrative
into sections such as:

- **The Early Years:** Reflect on your childhood and formative experiences, noting both the challenges and the moments of care or
  inspiration.
- **Moments of Crisis:** Identify key events that challenged your emotional resilience, and describe not only the pain but also the lessons
  learned.

- **Turning Points:** Highlight the moments when you began to reclaim your power—when therapy, support, or personal insights began to shift your perspective.
- **Emergence of a New Self:** Describe how you are building a new narrative, one that honors your past while embracing the possibilities of the future.

This outline helps organize your experiences into a coherent story. It allows you to see the progression of your journey and provides a roadmap for further growth. As you fill in the details of each chapter, you create a narrative that is uniquely yours—one that captures the complexity of your experiences and the beauty of your resilience.

## Affirmations and Future Visioning

In the process of rewriting your story, it's also important to envision the future you desire. Affirmations are a simple yet powerful way to reinforce this new narrative. Write affirmations that speak to your strengths and future aspirations, such as:

- "I am more than my struggles—I am a resilient, creative, and compassionate person."
- "Each challenge I overcome is a step toward a brighter, more empowered future."
- "My story is my own, and I have the power to shape it with hope and courage."

Pair these affirmations with visualization exercises. Close your eyes and imagine the life you want to live—a life where your narrative is defined not by pain but by growth, connection, and self-compassion. Let this vision inspire you to take concrete steps toward making that future a reality.

## Integrating Narrative Healing into Daily Life

The transformative power of narrative healing extends beyond solitary reflection or creative projects—it can be woven into the fabric of your daily life. Here are some strategies to help you integrate these practices consistently:

### Daily Reflection Time

Set aside a few minutes each day for quiet reflection. This could be part of a morning routine where you read a favorite affirmation or review a short journal entry from the day before. Regular reflection reinforces your evolving narrative and keeps you connected to your inner self.

### Sharing Your Journey

Consider joining a writing group, support group, or online forum where you can share your experiences and read about others' journeys. The act of sharing and listening can reinforce that your narrative is part of a larger tapestry of human experience. It also creates opportunities for mutual support and inspiration.

### Revisiting and Revising Your Narrative

Your narrative is not a fixed document—it evolves over time. Periodically revisit your journal, life story outline, or creative projects. Reflect on how your perspective has shifted and what new insights have emerged. Allow yourself the freedom to revise and expand your narrative as you grow. This ongoing process of reflection and revision can serve as a powerful reminder of your resilience and progress.

## The Ripple Effect of Personal Stories

When you heal through narrative, your story has the potential to reach far beyond your own life. By sharing your experiences, you not only empower yourself but also contribute to a broader cultural shift. Personal stories challenge the stigma and misunderstanding that often surround BPD. They humanize the clinical labels and offer hope to others who may be struggling in silence.

Memoirs like *Girl, Interrupted* have had a profound impact by revealing the real-life complexities behind mental health diagnoses. When you share your own narrative, you add another voice to the chorus calling for understanding, compassion, and change. Your story can help others see that while the journey may be fraught with challenges, it is also filled with beauty, resilience, and the possibility for renewal.

## Overcoming Barriers to Sharing Your Story

Sharing your personal narrative can feel vulnerable, and it's natural to have reservations. The fear of judgment, rejection, or further stigma can be powerful obstacles. However, it is important to recognize that your voice matters. Every story, when told with honesty and courage, has the power to heal both the teller and the listener.

### *Building a Safe Environment*

Before sharing your story publicly, consider creating a safe space where you feel supported. This might be a trusted circle of friends, a therapy group, or an online community dedicated to mental health. Start small by sharing excerpts of your narrative and gauge the response. Positive, empathetic feedback can bolster your confidence and encourage you to open up further.

## Setting Boundaries in Sharing

Remember that you control your narrative. It is perfectly acceptable to share only what you feel comfortable with. You can set boundaries regarding what parts of your story remain private and what you choose to share. As you become more confident in your voice, you may find that the act of sharing is itself a healing process, gradually diminishing the power of shame and self-doubt.

## Final Reflections on Narrative Healing

The journey of healing through narrative is a testament to the power of storytelling to transform pain into purpose. By embracing your personal story—its twists, turns, challenges, and triumphs—you reclaim control over your identity. Your narrative is not defined solely by your struggles with BPD; it is enriched by your resilience, creativity, and the unique insights you bring to the world.

Every word you write, every experience you share, and every reflection you engage in is a step toward healing. In rewriting your story, you not only honor your past but also chart a course for a future filled with possibility. The process may be challenging, and there may be moments when revisiting painful memories feels overwhelming. Yet, it is in these moments that the true power of narrative shines through—transforming wounds into wisdom and fear into hope.

May this chapter serve as an invitation to explore your own narrative with curiosity and compassion. Embrace the power of your story, knowing that every chapter, every line, is an integral part of the beautiful tapestry that is your life. As you continue on your journey, remember that healing is not about erasing the past but about integrating it into a larger narrative that celebrates who you are—resilient, empowered, and undeniably unique.

In the next chapter, we will explore how to build a supportive network and find mentors who can guide you along this transformative journey. Until then, take time to honor your narrative. Write, create, and share your story with pride, for it is through our stories that we not only heal ourselves but also light the way for others.

Embrace your voice, and let your story be a beacon of hope and strength in a world that needs to hear it.

# 10

# Building a Support Network – Finding Allies and Mentors

Healing from Borderline Personality Disorder (BPD) is not a journey that should be taken alone. While the process of self-discovery and self-acceptance is deeply personal, it is also shaped by the relationships we cultivate. A strong support network—a group of people who validate, encourage, and understand you—can be a crucial source of strength, especially during challenging times. In this chapter, we will explore how to identify, nurture, and maintain supportive relationships, including friends, family, professional mentors, and peer groups. We will also address the challenges that come with finding the right support and provide strategies for building meaningful connections that empower you to thrive.

## Why a Support Network Matters

Living with BPD often means experiencing intense emotions, fluctuating self-image, and difficulties in interpersonal relationships. These challenges can make it hard to reach out, especially when fear of abandonment or rejection is at play. However, a strong support system can help counter these struggles in several ways:

- **Validation:** Supportive people remind you that your feelings are real and that your experiences matter. They don't dismiss or belittle your emotions.
- **Perspective:** When emotions feel overwhelming, trusted allies can offer a more balanced perspective, helping you see the bigger picture rather than reacting impulsively.
- **Encouragement:** The right people will celebrate your progress and remind you of your strengths when you feel discouraged.
- **Accountability:** Having a support network can also keep you accountable in your healing journey, whether that means practicing DBT skills, attending therapy, or making healthy choices.

Building a supportive network is an investment in your well-being, and while it takes effort, the rewards are invaluable.

## Identifying Supportive People in Your Life

The first step in building a strong support network is identifying who in your life provides genuine support versus who may be reinforcing unhealthy patterns. Relationships fall on a spectrum—some are healing, some are neutral, and some may be harmful. It's essential to reflect on who brings out the best in you and who leaves you feeling drained or invalidated.

### Recognizing Healthy vs. Unhealthy Relationships

**Healthy Relationships:**

- Are based on mutual respect and understanding.

- Allow for open and honest communication.
- Involve emotional support without judgment.
- Encourage personal growth rather than dependency.

**Unhealthy Relationships:**

- Involve emotional manipulation, guilt-tripping, or constant criticism.
- Make you feel anxious, insecure, or like you have to "earn" love.
- Create cycles of toxicity where past wounds are reopened instead of healed.

It can be difficult to walk away from relationships that are unhealthy, especially when fear of abandonment is a major factor in BPD. However, prioritizing your well-being means surrounding yourself with people who uplift and support you rather than those who deepen your struggles.

## Types of Supportive Relationships

A healthy support network consists of different types of relationships, each playing a unique role in your life.

### 1. Close Friends and Family

Family members and long-term friends can be pillars of support—if they are willing to understand your experience. Educating loved ones about BPD can help them be more empathetic and patient. Some ways to strengthen these relationships include:

- Sharing resources such as books or articles about BPD.
- Encouraging open conversations about how they can best support

you.

- Setting clear boundaries to ensure that the relationship remains balanced.

However, if certain family members are unsupportive or trigger distress, it's okay to maintain distance. Healing does not require keeping relationships that are detrimental to your mental health.

## 2. Support Groups and Peer Networks

Connecting with others who share similar experiences can be incredibly validating. Support groups, whether in-person or online, provide a space to:

- Share struggles without fear of judgment.
- Exchange coping strategies and personal experiences.
- Find encouragement and hope in others' progress.

Many online communities, such as Facebook groups, Reddit forums, and mental health advocacy groups, offer peer support. However, it's important to choose spaces that promote healing rather than reinforce negative behaviors.

## 3. Therapists and Mental Health Professionals

Therapists, psychologists, and psychiatrists play a crucial role in guiding you through the complexities of BPD. A therapist trained in Dialectical Behavior Therapy (DBT) can provide structured tools for emotional regulation, distress tolerance, and interpersonal effectiveness. Finding a good therapist may take time, but it's worth the effort. If cost is a barrier, consider:

- Sliding scale therapy options.
- Community mental health centers.
- Online therapy platforms like BetterHelp or Talkspace.

## 4. Mentors and Role Models

Mentors can be invaluable in your growth. A mentor doesn't have to be a mental health professional; they can be someone you admire for their resilience, wisdom, or personal journey. A mentor can provide:

- Encouragement and advice during difficult times.
- Practical guidance for achieving personal or professional goals.
- A reminder that healing and growth are possible.

Some people find mentors in professional settings, creative communities, or advocacy groups. The key is to seek out people whose values align with your own and who model the kind of emotional stability and growth you aspire to.

## Strategies for Building a Support Network

Once you've identified who in your life provides positive support, the next step is actively cultivating these relationships.

## 1. Strengthening Existing Relationships

- **Be honest about your needs.** Let trusted friends and family know how they can support you. For example, you might say, "When I'm feeling overwhelmed, I just need someone to listen without offering solutions."
- **Show appreciation.** Supportive people need affirmation too. Ex-

pressing gratitude strengthens the relationship and fosters mutual respect.

- **Communicate boundaries.** If certain topics or behaviors trigger distress, express your boundaries clearly. Healthy relationships respect those limits.

## 2. Expanding Your Circle

If your current social circle feels limited, consider:

- **Attending support groups or mental health meetups.** Many communities offer in-person and online support groups for individuals with BPD.
- **Engaging in interest-based communities.** Whether it's a writing group, art class, or fitness club, connecting over shared passions can foster meaningful relationships.
- **Volunteering or joining advocacy groups.** Working toward a cause you believe in can introduce you to like-minded individuals who share your values.

## 3. Knowing When to Let Go

Not every relationship is meant to last. If a connection consistently brings negativity into your life, it may be time to let it go. Ending toxic relationships is difficult, but it's a form of self-care. Consider:

- Slowly distancing yourself if cutting ties abruptly feels too overwhelming.
- Seeking support from a therapist to navigate the process.
- Reminding yourself that protecting your peace is not selfish—it's necessary for healing.

## Overcoming Barriers to Seeking Support

For many women with BPD, seeking support can feel daunting. The fear of rejection, mistrust of others, or belief that you must "handle everything alone" can become barriers to reaching out. Here's how to navigate these fears:

### 1. Challenge the Fear of Burdening Others

It's common to feel like your struggles might be too much for others to handle. However, healthy relationships involve give and take. Those who genuinely care about you want to be there for you.

### 2. Build Trust Gradually

If past betrayals have made it difficult to trust, take small steps. Share little things first, and see how someone responds before opening up more. Trust is built over time.

### 3. Practice Receiving Support

Receiving kindness and validation can feel uncomfortable if you're used to self-reliance. Try to accept support, even if it feels foreign. Letting others help can be an act of courage.

### 4. Seek Professional Guidance

If opening up feels impossible, a therapist can provide tools to help you navigate trust issues and develop healthier relationship patterns.

## The Power of a Supportive Community

A strong support network doesn't just help in difficult moments—it enhances your life in every way. When you surround yourself with people who uplift and understand you, healing becomes a shared journey rather than an isolated struggle.

- **You feel seen.** Your emotions and experiences are validated, reducing the loneliness that often accompanies BPD.
- **You gain perspective.** Others help you navigate challenges by offering different viewpoints and encouragement.
- **You grow together.** A good support system challenges you to be your best self while offering unconditional love and patience.

## Final Thoughts

Building a support network is one of the most empowering steps you can take in your healing journey. It requires effort, patience, and sometimes the courage to let go of what no longer serves you. But in the end, the relationships you cultivate will provide strength, encouragement, and a sense of belonging.

You do not have to navigate BPD alone. There are people—whether friends, therapists, mentors, or peers—who will walk this journey with you. By seeking and nurturing those connections, you create a foundation of support that allows you to grow, heal, and thrive.

In the next chapter, we will explore tools for long-term transformation—how to integrate the skills you've learned into everyday life and continue your journey toward lasting emotional well-being.

# 11

# Tools for Transformation – Empowerment Strategies and Long-Term Healing

As we move deeper into the journey of healing from Borderline Personality Disorder (BPD), it's important to shift the focus from short-term coping mechanisms to long-term empowerment. While therapy, medication, and support networks play crucial roles, true transformation requires building sustainable strategies that empower you to reclaim your life, define your identity beyond your diagnosis, and create a future grounded in emotional balance, resilience, and self-compassion.

This chapter will explore tools for long-term transformation, including habit formation, emotional mastery, goal-setting, and self-empowerment techniques. By integrating these strategies, you can move beyond survival mode and begin to thrive.

## The Shift from Healing to Thriving

For many women with BPD, life can feel like a constant cycle of emotional crises, relationship struggles, and internal battles. In the early stages of recovery, the focus is often on damage control—learning to regulate emotions, avoiding harmful behaviors, and navigating relationships more effectively. But healing is about more than just managing symptoms; it's about stepping into your power and reclaiming control over your life.

Moving from healing to thriving requires:

- **Building emotional stability that lasts beyond therapy sessions.**
- **Cultivating self-confidence and self-trust.**
- **Developing meaningful goals and working toward personal growth.**
- **Shaping a life that aligns with your passions, values, and dreams.**

This transition is not linear, and setbacks are inevitable. However, by adopting long-term transformation strategies, you can ensure that each setback becomes a stepping stone rather than a roadblock.

# 1. Mastering Emotional Resilience

## *Understanding Emotional Regulation as a Lifestyle*

Emotional regulation is not just a DBT skill to be used in moments of distress—it is a lifelong practice that enhances overall well-being. To cultivate emotional resilience, focus on:

- **Mindfulness as a daily habit:** Integrate mindfulness into daily activities such as eating, walking, or commuting. The more present you become in everyday life, the easier it is to stay grounded during emotional storms.
- **Regular emotional check-ins:** Develop the habit of asking yourself, "How am I feeling right now?" Recognizing emotions early allows you to manage them before they spiral.
- **Processing emotions healthily:** Engage in creative outlets like

journaling, painting, or dancing to express emotions constructively rather than suppressing them.

## Building a Resilient Mindset

Resilience is not about avoiding emotional pain but about learning how to bounce back. You can strengthen resilience by:

- **Reframing setbacks as learning experiences:** Instead of seeing struggles as failures, ask, "What can I learn from this?"
- **Practicing self-soothing techniques:** Engage in deep breathing, progressive muscle relaxation, or grounding exercises when feeling overwhelmed.
- **Developing distress tolerance:** Accept that discomfort is a part of life and focus on riding the wave rather than resisting it.

# 2. Habit Formation for Long-Term Change

One of the most effective ways to create lasting transformation is through habit formation. Small, consistent actions shape our daily lives and, over time, become second nature.

## The Science of Habit Formation

According to Charles Duhigg's *The Power of Habit*, habits are formed through a three-step loop:

1. **Cue:** A trigger that initiates the behavior (e.g., feeling stressed).
2. **Routine:** The action you take in response (e.g., practicing mindfulness instead of self-harming).
3. **Reward:** The benefit you gain from the action (e.g., feeling calmer

and more in control).

By replacing unhealthy coping mechanisms with healthier routines, you rewire your brain to respond differently to emotional triggers.

### Practical Strategies for Creating Positive Habits

- **Start small:** Focus on one habit at a time, such as drinking water when feeling overwhelmed or taking a five-minute break to breathe before reacting impulsively.
- **Use habit stacking:** Attach new habits to existing ones (e.g., practicing gratitude every morning before brushing your teeth).
- **Track progress:** Keep a habit tracker or journal to stay motivated and monitor your growth.
- **Reward yourself:** Celebrate small victories to reinforce positive behavior.

## 3. Defining and Achieving Personal Goals

### From Survival Mode to Purpose-Driven Living

BPD can often make life feel chaotic, leaving little room for long-term planning. However, once you move beyond crisis management, setting meaningful goals can give your life direction and purpose.

### How to Set Empowering Goals

Use the SMART goal framework to create goals that are:

- **Specific:** Clearly define what you want to achieve.
- **Measurable:** Track progress and celebrate milestones.

- **Achievable:** Set realistic expectations to avoid frustration.
- **Relevant:** Align goals with your passions and values.
- **Time-bound:** Establish deadlines to stay motivated.

For example, instead of saying, "I want to feel better," a SMART goal would be:

"I will practice mindfulness for five minutes every morning for the next 30 days."

## Breaking Goals into Actionable Steps

Large goals can feel overwhelming, so break them down into smaller steps. If your goal is to improve your relationships, start by:

1. Practicing one new communication skill each week.
2. Scheduling time to nurture existing friendships.
3. Seeking support in therapy or a support group.

By focusing on small, consistent actions, you make long-term change more manageable.

## 4. Developing Self-Compassion and Confidence

### Overcoming Self-Criticism

Many women with BPD struggle with intense self-judgment, often feeling "not good enough." However, self-compassion is one of the most powerful tools for transformation.

- **Practice positive self-talk:** Replace self-criticism with affirmations such as "I am learning and growing every day."

- **Acknowledge progress:** Reflect on how far you've come rather than focusing on where you fall short.
- **Forgive yourself:** Understand that healing is a process, and mistakes do not define you.

## Embracing Your Strengths

BPD often heightens sensitivity, creativity, and intuition—qualities that can be harnessed as strengths. Recognizing these strengths can boost confidence and reshape your self-perception.

- **Celebrate your empathy:** Your deep emotional understanding allows you to connect with others meaningfully.
- **Use creativity as a tool:** Channel intense emotions into writing, music, or visual art.
- **Acknowledge your resilience:** Every challenge you've overcome is proof of your strength.

## 5. Cultivating a Lifestyle That Supports Long-Term Stability

Long-term healing requires aligning your lifestyle with your mental and emotional well-being.

## 1. Prioritizing Physical Health

- **Regular exercise:** Activities like yoga, dancing, or walking can help regulate emotions and reduce stress.
- **Balanced nutrition:** A well-nourished body supports a well-balanced mind. Avoid excessive caffeine, sugar, and processed foods.
- **Consistent sleep schedule:** Sleep deprivation can intensify emo-

tional instability, so establish a bedtime routine that promotes restfulness.

## 2. Creating a Structured Daily Routine

A lack of structure can contribute to emotional instability. Establishing routines helps create predictability and stability.

- **Morning routine:** Start the day with mindfulness, journaling, or light movement.
- **Evening routine:** Wind down with relaxation techniques, gratitude reflection, or reading.
- **Time blocking:** Set aside dedicated time for work, self-care, socializing, and rest.

## 3. Engaging in Meaningful Activities

Engaging in activities that bring joy and fulfillment is crucial for long-term healing.

- **Volunteer work:** Helping others can provide a sense of purpose and connection.
- **Pursuing hobbies:** Whether it's playing an instrument, gardening, or painting, hobbies create space for personal expression.
- **Learning new skills:** Expanding your knowledge fosters confidence and personal growth.

## Final Reflections: Becoming the Architect of Your Future

Healing from BPD is not about reaching a final destination—it's about continuously evolving into the best version of yourself. By implementing empowerment strategies, you can move beyond managing symptoms and step into a life filled with meaning, stability, and fulfillment.

As you integrate these tools into your daily routine, remember:

- **You have the power to reshape your story.**
- **Your emotions are part of you, but they do not define you.**
- **Every small step forward is a victory.**

The journey of transformation is lifelong, but with each mindful choice, you are building a future grounded in resilience, self-acceptance, and empowerment.

In the final chapter, we will explore what it means to truly live beyond BPD—embracing a life of authenticity, purpose, and unshakable self-worth. Until then, trust in your progress, honor your growth, and know that you are capable of incredible transformation.

# 12

# Beyond the Diagnosis – Embracing a Life of Authenticity and Fulfillment

The journey of healing from Borderline Personality Disorder (BPD) is not simply about managing symptoms—it is about reclaiming your life. It is about moving beyond the constraints of a diagnosis and stepping into a future where you define yourself not by past struggles but by your resilience, growth, and authenticity.

This final chapter is an invitation to embrace life fully, to move past fear, and to step into a version of yourself that is grounded, empowered, and free. Together, we will explore what it means to truly live beyond BPD, cultivate self-acceptance, and create a life filled with meaning, purpose, and fulfillment.

## Redefining Yourself Beyond BPD

For many women with BPD, the diagnosis can feel all-encompassing. It can shape the way you see yourself and how others perceive you. However, BPD is not your identity—it is simply one part of your story. The goal of healing is not to erase this part of yourself but to integrate it in a way that allows you to thrive.

## Who Are You Without the Label?

When you think about yourself outside of BPD, who do you see?

- What qualities define you beyond your emotional struggles?
- What dreams and aspirations have been buried beneath self-doubt?
- What passions and interests light you up inside?

Healing is about rediscovering the parts of yourself that were overshadowed by pain and reclaiming the joy, curiosity, and individuality that make you who you are.

## Moving from "Broken" to Whole

Many women with BPD internalize the idea that they are "too much" or "not enough"—that they are somehow broken. But you are not broken. You are evolving. Every challenge you have faced has contributed to the depth of your empathy, your strength, and your ability to connect deeply with the world around you.

Reframing your self-perception is key to living beyond BPD. Instead of focusing on what is "wrong" with you, shift your mindset to acknowledge what is **right** about you:

- Your ability to feel deeply is a gift.
- Your sensitivity makes you a compassionate and intuitive person.
- Your struggles have given you a level of resilience that many will never understand.

By embracing all aspects of yourself—including the difficult emotions— you step into a place of wholeness rather than fragmentation.

# Living Authentically – Embracing Your True Self

## What Does It Mean to Live Authentically?

Living authentically means embracing who you are, unapologetically. It means honoring your emotions, needs, and desires without fear of judgment. It is about making choices based on what aligns with your values rather than what is expected of you.

For many women with BPD, the fear of rejection leads to people-pleasing, masking, or adjusting one's personality to fit different situations. While adaptability is a strength, it should never come at the cost of losing your true self.

Authentic living requires:

- **Honesty with yourself and others.**
- **Setting boundaries that protect your emotional well-being.**
- **Pursuing passions and interests that resonate with your soul.**
- **Letting go of relationships, environments, or beliefs that no longer serve you.**

## Practicing Self-Acceptance

Self-acceptance is not about liking yourself all the time—it is about recognizing that you are worthy, regardless of your imperfections.

- **Affirm Your Worth Daily:** Use affirmations such as, "I am enough just as I am," or "I deserve kindness, from myself and others."
- **Let Go of the Need for External Validation:** True confidence comes from within. Seeking approval from others will always leave you feeling dependent on their opinions.
- **Celebrate Your Progress:** Healing is a journey. Take time to

acknowledge how far you have come, even if the steps feel small.

The more you practice self-acceptance, the more comfortable you become with yourself—and the easier it is to live authentically.

## Finding Purpose and Meaning in Life

### The Importance of a Meaningful Life

A significant part of healing is shifting from survival mode to **purpose-driven living**. When your life is filled with meaning, you are less likely to feel consumed by emotional turbulence. Purpose gives you a reason to wake up each day with intention.

### How to Discover Your Purpose

1. **Reflect on What Brings You Joy:** What activities make you lose track of time? What moments make you feel most alive?
2. **Consider Your Strengths:** Your struggles have given you unique insights. How can you use them to help others or contribute to the world?
3. **Explore Different Avenues:** Try volunteering, creative pursuits, or learning new skills. Experimentation is key to discovering your passions.
4. **Define Your Core Values:** What principles do you want to guide your life? Honesty, compassion, creativity, adventure? Align your daily choices with these values.

Purpose does not have to be grand—it can be found in the small, everyday moments of connection, kindness, and self-expression.

## Creating a Life You Love

Once you have begun redefining yourself, embracing authenticity, and finding purpose, the next step is to **actively create a life that reflects your true self**.

### 1. Design Your Ideal Daily Routine

How you spend your days is how you spend your life. Small daily choices shape the bigger picture.

- **Morning Rituals:** Start your day with mindfulness, gratitude, or journaling to set a positive tone.
- **Work or Passion Projects:** Engage in work that feels meaningful, whether it's a job, hobby, or creative endeavor.
- **Self-Care Practices:** Prioritize physical, emotional, and mental well-being.
- **Evening Wind-Down:** Reflect on your day, unwind with relaxation techniques, and set intentions for tomorrow.

### 2. Surround Yourself with People Who Uplift You

The relationships in your life should reflect your growth and values. Surround yourself with people who:

- Encourage your dreams.
- Respect your boundaries.
- Bring positivity and balance into your life.
- Accept you for who you are.

Let go of toxic relationships that drain your energy or make you feel small.

## 3. Continue Growing and Learning

Healing is an ongoing journey. Keep expanding your mind and experiences by:

- Reading books that inspire personal growth.
- Trying new activities outside of your comfort zone.
- Seeking out therapy or mentorship when needed.
- Engaging in self-reflection regularly.

Transformation is continuous. The person you are becoming will continue to evolve.

## Embracing the Future with Confidence

### You Are Not Your Past

No matter what you have been through, **your past does not define you**. The mistakes, pain, and struggles you have faced are chapters in your story, not the entire book. You have the power to write new chapters— ones filled with joy, love, adventure, and self-acceptance.

### The Courage to Live Boldly

Living beyond BPD requires courage. It means taking risks, opening yourself to new experiences, and allowing yourself to believe in a future that is bigger than your past pain.

- **Dare to dream big.**

- **Allow yourself to experience happiness without fear.**
- **Trust that you are capable of love and connection.**
- **Believe in your ability to handle life's challenges.**

## You Are Enough

At the heart of this journey, the most important lesson is this: **you are enough, just as you are.** Not when you're "fixed," not when you've "earned" love—right now, in this moment.

The road beyond BPD is one of empowerment, self-acceptance, and transformation. It is about stepping into a life that is truly yours, filled with meaning, passion, and authenticity.

As you close this book, know that this is not the end of your journey—it is just the beginning. **You are free to create a life that reflects the depth, beauty, and resilience of who you truly are.**

**Live boldly. Live fully. Live as the person you were always meant to be.**